DOPPELGÄNGER

'Femi Oyebode has written an incredible book on the doppelgänger phenomenon across history, film, literature, and medicine. As a poet, scholar of medical humanities, clinician scientist, and internationally pre-eminent psychopathologist, I can think of no one better [than Professor Oyebode] to take on this important synthesis and novel argument across multiple academic disciplines. The conclusions of this rich monograph are striking and important: the illusion of the virtual other is a necessary consequence of our existence as experiencing embodied beings tempted by a Cartesian dualism, and the apparent splitting of self and body. I recommend this book not only to clinicians and neuroscientists, but also to cultural historians, literary and film scholars, and philosophers. I have no doubt that the book will impact on my own clinical practice with patients who are frightened by seeing their own doubles.'

*Professor **Matthew Broome**, Chair in Psychiatry and Youth Mental Health, University of Birmingham, UK*

DOPPELGÄNGER

Analysing 'Doubles' across, Antiquity, Fiction, Film, Psychopathology, and Neuroscience

Femi Oyebode

University of Birmingham

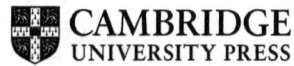

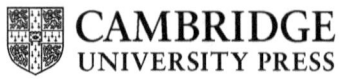

Shaftesbury Road, Cambridge CB2 8EA, United Kingdom

One Liberty Plaza, 20th Floor, New York, NY 10006, USA

477 Williamstown Road, Port Melbourne, VIC 3207, Australia

314–321, 3rd Floor, Plot 3, Splendor Forum, Jasola District Centre,
New Delhi – 110025, India

103 Penang Road, #05–06/07, Visioncrest Commercial, Singapore 238467

Cambridge University Press is part of Cambridge University Press & Assessment,
a department of the University of Cambridge.

We share the University's mission to contribute to society through the pursuit of
education, learning and research at the highest international levels of excellence.

www.cambridge.org
Information on this title: www.cambridge.org/9781009305761

DOI: 10.1017/9781009305730

© The Royal College of Psychiatrists 2025

This publication is in copyright. Subject to statutory exception and to the provisions of relevant collective licensing agreements, no reproduction of any part may take place without the written permission of Cambridge University Press & Assessment.

When citing this work, please include a reference to the DOI 10.1017/9781009305730

First published 2025

A catalogue record for this publication is available from the British Library

A Cataloging-in-Publication data record for this book is available from the Library of Congress

ISBN 978-1-009-30576-1 Paperback

Cambridge University Press & Assessment has no responsibility for the persistence or accuracy of URLs for external or third-party internet websites referred to in this publication and does not guarantee that any content on such websites is, or will remain, accurate or appropriate.

Every effort has been made in preparing this book to provide accurate and up-to-date information that is in accord with accepted standards and practice at the time of publication. Although case histories are drawn from actual cases, every effort has been made to disguise the identities of the individuals involved. Nevertheless, the authors, editors, and publishers can make no warranties that the information contained herein is totally free from error, not least because clinical standards are constantly changing through research and regulation. The authors, editors, and publishers therefore disclaim all liability for direct or consequential damages resulting from the use of material contained in this book. Readers are strongly advised to pay careful attention to information provided by the manufacturer of any drugs or equipment that they plan to use.

For Oyinlola and Akintokunbo

Contents

1	Introduction	1
2	The Double in Antiquity	18
3	The Double as Other in the Novel	33
4	The Double as Duality in Fiction	78
5	Implicit Double in Fiction	88
6	The Double in Film	106
7	The Double in Clinical Psychopathology	127
8	The Double in Neuroscience	142
9	The Ultimate Illusion: Understanding Embodiment and the Self	152
References		164
Index		168

CHAPTER 1

Introduction

The same august presence, the same grace of movement, the same intelligent eyes, the same broad forehead, the divine smile; the only difference was that her body seemed fuller and more youthful...

(E. T. A. Hoffmann 1776–1822)

The term doppelgänger was first used by Jean Paul Richter in his novel *Siebenkäs* published in 1796. Jean Paul Richter (Figure 1.1), also known as Jean Paul, was a prominent German writer and humorist of the late eighteenth and early nineteenth centuries. He was born on 21 March 1763, in Wunsiedel, Bavaria, and is best known for his humorous and imaginative novels. Richter's works often combined satire, sentimentality, and whimsy, engaging readers with his wit and wordplay. His other notable works include *Titan* (1800–1803) and *Flegeljahre* (1804–1805). Richter's writing style and inventive language had a significant influence on subsequent generations of German authors. He died on 4 November 1825 in Bayreuth.

The term doppelgänger translates as 'double walker'. *Siebenkäs* is a bildungsroman, a type of novel that focuses on the psychological and moral growth of the main character. The novel follows the story of Leibgeber, an impoverished and mischievous young man who is constantly getting into trouble. Despite his flaws, he is loved by the people around him for his wit and humour. The plot of the novel revolves around Leibgeber's attempts to improve his financial and social status. Along the way, he encounters many obstacles and experiences various emotional and psychological trials, which shape his character and help him to grow and mature. One of the central themes of the novel is the idea of the 'doppelgänger', or double, which Richter introduces as a motif to explore the concept of identity and the duality of human nature. Throughout the novel, Leibgeber grapples with the

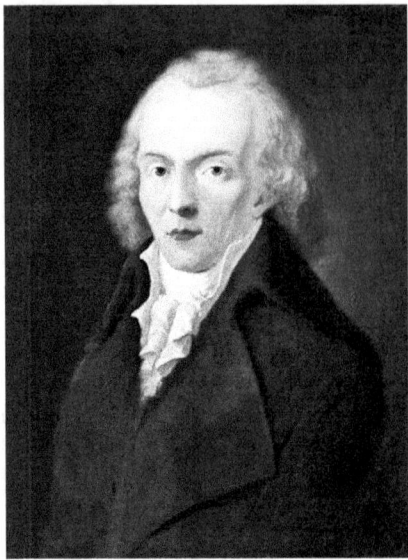

Figure 1.1 Jean Paul Richter 1763–1825 (Public domain)

idea of who he is and what his place in the world is, and the doppelgänger serves as a symbol of the different parts of his personality.

Richter's interest in doppelganger may itself derive from his personal experience. He wrote,

> Never shall I forget that inward occurrence, till now narrated to no mortal, wherein I witnessed the birth of my Self-consciousness, of which I can still give the place and time. One forenoon, I was standing, a very young child, in the outer door, and looking leftward at the stack of fuel wood, – when all at once the internal vision, – I am a Me (och bin win Och), came like a flash from heaven before me, and in gleaming light ever afterwards continued: then had my Me, for the first time, seen itself, and for ever. (Richter, 1863)

In the novel, the protagonist, Siebenkäs, meets with his double, Leibgeber, at his [Siebenkäs] wedding, and this encounter is described as follows:

> So singular an alliance between two singular souls is not often seen. The same contempt for the ennobled childish nonsense of life; the same enmity to the mean, with every indulgence to the little; the same indignation

against dishonest selfishness; the same love of laughing in the beautiful madhouse of earth; the same deafness to the voice of the world, but not of honor; – these were but the more superficial traits of resemblance that constituted them one soul assigned to two bodies. Neither do I take much into account that they were foster-brothers in their studies, and were nursed by the same sciences, including even the law; inasmuch as similarity of studies is often the best dissolvent and precipitant of friendship. Nor was it simply the want of resemblance, which, as an opposite pole, decided their attraction, was more ready to forgive, to punish; the former was more to be compared to a satire of Horace, the latter to a ballad of Aristophanes, with its unpoetical and poetical dissonances; but like girls who, when they become friends, love to wear the same dress, so did their souls wear exactly the same frock-coat and morning dress of life; I mean, two bodies, with the same cupfuls and collars, of the same color, button-holes, trimmings, and cut. Both had the same brightness of eye, the same sallowness of face, the same height, and the same meagreness; for the phenomenon of similarity of feature is more common than is generally believed, believed, being only remarked when some prince or great man casts a bodily reflection. I wish, therefore, that Leibgeber had not limped, which somewhat distinguished him from Siebenkäs, especially as the latter had cleverly scratched and burnt away, by means of a living toad which he had caused to die on the spot, a mark which, on his side, might have distinguished him from Leibgeber. This mark was a pyramidal mole near the left ear, in the shape of a triangle, or of the zodiacal light, or of a turned-up comet's tail, or, more correctly still, of an ass's ear. (Richter, 1863, pp. 1024–1039)

So was born the modern tradition of doppelganger, a fictional character who is both physically and psychologically identical, save for minor anomalies. As Paul Meehan (2017) puts it in his book *The Ghost of One's Self: Doppelgangers in Mystery, Horror and Science Fiction Films*, 'It's you but it's not you. It's an inverse mirror image, a double, an alter ego, a simulacrum, a clone. It's your shadow self, your evil twin, your most significant other, your dark half. It's your doppelganger' (p. 3).

The term doppelgänger has now come to stand for the existence of a double of a living person. The double is conceived of as an exact but sometimes invisible replica of a person, sometimes of a bird or a beast.

This belief has a long antiquity and is a widespread belief among cultural groups the world over. Other words that refer to related concepts include alter ego, familiar, fetch, and wraith. In ancient Egyptian mythology, the *ka* was seen as a concrete spirit double, and among the Yoruba, in West Africa, it is believed that everyone has an *ikeji*, an unseen double. In Norse mythology, *vardogers* are ghostly doubles that mimic the actions and behaviours of their living counterparts, and in Celtic culture, *a fetch* is an identical twin that is said to appear at the moment of one's death. In the Icelandic sagas, a fetch (*fylgja*) is literally someone that accompanies, a personal spirit that was closely attached to families and individuals, and often symbolized the fate that people were born with. If it appeared to an individual or others close to him or her, it would often signal the impending doom of that person. Fetches could take various forms, sometimes appearing in the shape of an animal as exemplified in Philip Pullman's *His Dark Materials* where some of his characters have visible demons that are animal-shaped, who accompany them everywhere. In this account of fetches, detachment of these animal forms leaves their human counterparts as empty shells.

Icelandic fetches too tend to be corporeal. In *Eirich the Red's Saga*, Sigrid, who was already ill, went to the outhouse and remarked, 'All those who are dead are standing there before the door'; among them I recognise your husband Thorstein and myself as well. How horrible to see it! ... 'Before morning came she was dead' (Eiríksson, 1997, p. 663; Smilely, 2005).

It is, perhaps, not surprising that we have a preoccupation with the notion of duplication as there is a duality represented in our bodies: we have two upper and lower limbs, two eyes, two ears, two nostrils, two testicles, and so on. Even those parts of our bodies that appear singular, like our faces, are in two symmetrical halves and our brains are also in two halves. And to complicate matters, our limbs that look superficially identical are, on closer scrutiny, marginally different in size and proportion, as are the two halves of our faces. This gives the impression that the apparent identity of our duplicated organs itself conceals distinctness and difference. Hence, notions of the double, of doppelgänger, work on this assumption of another who is identical but potentially different – different either in physique, personality, or psychology.

Yet, our subjective experience of who we are is that of a singular, unique, unified, and embodied self. This sense of being a single and coherent self, one that is consistent and unified over time and that has a distinct identity, a biography, and physiognomy, a uniqueness, is one of the most profound and fundamental subjective experiences that we all have. I mean by this the feeling of having been oneself, for as long as one can remember, integrated into a recognizable and identifiable body, despite marked changes attributable to physical development and ageing, and to personal growth and emotional maturation.

This subjective experience of a unified and unique self is foundational to who we all are. But it is built on the implicit notion that we experience ourselves as alive, as lively, and as vital. This sense of vitality is closely associated with the sense of being an active agent, one who initiates and executes actions and who has responsibility for these actions, who is distinct from other things and other beings, and who is aware of oneself and recognizes what is *myself* from what is *other*. And has this profound sense of singularity.

We could say that these characteristics of the self are the pillars on which our sense of self is built. More formally, these characteristics are referred to as awareness of unity of the self, awareness of identity of the self, awareness of vitality of the self, awareness of activity of the self, and awareness of boundaries of the self, respectively. They are formal, conceptual properties of the self. They are neither objective nor concrete properties since they do not derive from empirical science or observations. This is a way of saying that the term 'self' is merely a concept, a notion of what it is to be a person and not a thing. Nonetheless, even though the term is not empirically grounded, it is true that subjectively we experience ourselves in these ways, and that these ways of being are fundamental to our self-concept.

What is remarkable is that these characteristics of the self, namely that we are single, unique, and coherent over time, alive, active, and with a boundary that renders us distinct from other beings, seem so obvious, so self-evident that they form the background, implicit structure that makes our subjective experiences possible and comprehensible, at all. We rarely ever doubt these foundational characteristics of ourselves. It is only when these formal characteristics are somehow breached, when they are undermined by disease or functionally impaired, that we start to recognize the formal structures that make possible normal experiences. When we encounter the ways that these abnormalities are manifest within the clinical space, we are often surprised and intrigued, sometimes perplexed. We may see an individual who complains of seeing his exact double standing beside him, even if briefly. Or we may see a person who believes that he has an exact double acting in the world, who he has yet to meet, but who has advertised his existence by malicious acts committed in the name of the patient. Finally, we may see, even if rarely, a person who exhibits dual or multiple personalities and who inhabits the self-same body. Perhaps, less controversially, we may see people who have contradictory aspects of the self, individuals who, on the face of it, seem pleasant and genial but at other times vicious, callous, and murderous. These clinical scenarios prompt us to recognize, if not admit, that the subjective experiences or foundational beliefs that are so matter of fact, so implicit to how we conceive of our world, may in fact be more complex than we imagine. At the very least, these clinical scenarios set the stage for a re-evaluation of the ordinary ways that we structure our world. The possibility of separation of the self from the body, as an idea, as an experience, or as an experience that is verified by perception, disrupts the accepted ways of looking at the nature of the self, and its relationship to the body. And the possibility that there may be distinct and multiple personalities in a single body or indeed that there are contradictory aspects of the self that are not coherent or well-integrated raises questions about the nature of identity, and of the self too.

This book is about the nature of the double in all its various manifestations, from folklore to literature and cinema, and from clinical psychopathology to clinical neuroscience. The notions and concepts evident in folklore and literature, the actual experiences reported by patients in the clinic, and the experimental evidence from neuroscience all raise serious questions about how the mind and the self are understood in the philosophy of mind and how notions of the embodied self are described in cognitive neuroscience. The issues that the empirical evidence of the double, particularly as drawn from autoscopy, from the delusional misidentification syndromes, and from dissociative identity disorder (multiple personality disorder), raise for philosophy are profound, but they are equally profound for our understanding of what it is to be human.

INTRODUCTION

Concepts of Mind and Self

I want now to turn to some groundwork. I want to explore our current understanding of terms such as mind and self. The term 'mind' has come to stand for all that is peculiarly human. Our capacity for language, for conscious awareness, for music making, for mathematics, for formal logic, and for many more indefinable skills and aptitudes are understood as features of our mind. What is common to these capacities is that they are all examples of mental activity. We could also add that attention, memory, perception, emotion, volition, and affect are further examples of mental activity. I am here drawing attention to the degree to which the nature of mind is at the very least involved in our conception of ourselves as humans. This is to say that the nature of man, of the person, is intertwined with any description that we choose to give of mind. So, if it were to be shown that mind is solely a property of the brain and that a physical description exhausts all that there is to be known about mind, then a person would be no more than a material body, even if a complex material body. On the other hand, a description that grants the mind an existence independent of the brain would at the same time grant man a dimension that is free from the material. These matters are at the very heart of the subject of this book, namely how we can come to understand how it is possible for doubles to exist in the clinic. Are the experiences of doubles that we encounter in clinical psychiatry the only evidence of perturbations in neural circuitry, or do they tell us something more fundamental about the nature of mind, self, and their relationship to the material brain?

The distinction that I have been making is best addressed by Sergio Moravia (1995). He argues that the 'curious, old-fashioned problem of the relationship between mind and body ... raises several crucial questions with respect to knowledge in general and to man and his science'. He asks,

> a) can one posit something that *exists*, and yet at the same time is *non-physical* b) can physicalist knowledge give an adequate description and explanation of 'all that there is' ... or does something exist the cognition of which requires a knowledge which is independent of that provided by

the physical sciences? c) Do the rejection of 'soul' and the achievements by the bio- and neurosciences oblige us to hold that man is *nothing but body*? (Moravia, 1995, pp. 4–5, emphasis in original)

Moravia's thesis is that 'it is simply wrong to suppose that whatever is not encompassed by a directly or indirectly materialist monism is "inaccessible to human investigation". This would mean reducing human knowledge to solely *physical knowledge*' (p. 7). Moravia is sensitive to the fact that the solution to the mind–brain problem speaks to other problems in philosophy. And, specifically, that any description that privileges the physical over the psychological would in some way reduce man. For Moravia, 'the mental, and on its behalf psychological language, *speaks about man*' (p. 24) (all emphasis in the original). So, Moravia is echoing, albeit in a slightly different language, René Descartes's (1596–1650) theory, namely that we are ultimately thinking beings and that this aspect of us is not extended in length, width, or depth and is not dependent on the body for its existence but is nonetheless real. Descartes's influential theory of dualism argues for the undeniable existence of a thinking mind, one that is immaterial and non-physical. To summarize, Moravia's position is to resist any attempt to materialize or physicalize mind.

Another approach to understanding the nature of mind is that taken by Gilbert Ryle (1900–1976) (Ryle, 1949; 1990). His thesis is that the term 'mind' stands for the unity of all the processes and operations of the brain, including such relatively better understood processes as language, memory, and vision and lesser understood processes such as intentionality and consciousness. He accepts that in everyday use, the word 'mind' behaves sometimes as if mind is a place or a thing, but for Ryle this is simply a way of speaking. When we say 'I have something in mind', we are not referring to a specific place, or when we say 'I will work on it with my mind', we are not referring to an extra tool with which to solve a problem. For Ryle, 'mind' is simply a term that stands for all brain processes and operations. It is, in other words, a concept. It does not refer to a place, a thing, or a tool. It is not a function. If we were to ask if animals have minds, the answer would depend on our conception of animals. There would be no empirical test to validate the response. However, if one were to ask if animals have the use of language, this would be an empirical question with a possible empirical answer. This way of approaching the mind locates it in the same domain as other words like justice, freedom, hope, and so on.

The mind can be seen as distinct from and independent of the body or as no more than a concept. I will return to these issues later. But for now, what about the term 'self'? There is little doubt that, the way we use this term, it stands both for the subject of experience as well as the initiator of action. Galen Strawson (1997) describes the self as the sense that people have of themselves as being, specifically a mental presence, a mental someone, a conscious subject that has a certain character or personality, and that is distinct from all its particular experiences, thoughts, hopes, wishes, feelings, and so on. And that this connects with the feeling that their body is just a vehicle or vessel for the mental thing that they really are. This approach speaks to the everyday phenomenology of the self. But as with the term 'mind', the term 'self' can also be understood as a concept, only. Dave Hume (1711–1776) in *A Treatise of Human Nature* (Hume & Selby-Bigge, 1789) writes, 'What we call mind is nothing but a heap or collection of different perceptions, united together by certain relations, and suppos'd, tho' falsely, to be endowed with a perfect simplicity and identity' (p. 207).

In other words, Hume's position is that our observations of the world are theory impregnated, and that these theories are formed from habits of mind rather than logically derived. In *A Treatise of Human Nature*, Hume appears to take a phenomenologist approach:

> When I enter most intimately into what I call *myself*, I always stumble on some particular perception or other, of heat or cold, light or shade ... I never catch *myself* at any time without a perception, and never can observe anything but the perception. When my perceptions are remov'd for any time, as by sound sleep; so long am I insensible of *myself*, and may truly be said not to exist. (p. 252, emphasis in the original)

> The mind is a kind of theatre, where several perceptions successively make their appearance ... There is properly no simplicity in it at one time, nor identity ... There are successive perceptions only, that constitute the mind; nor have we the most distant notion of the place, where these scenes are represented, or the materials of which it is compoms'd. (p. 253)

For Hume, the self is an agglomeration of perceptions, the centre of experience but nonetheless an illusory centre of perception in which the sense of unity and identity are fictitious. A clear objection to Hume already resides in the opening line of his famous sentence, 'When I enter most intimately into what I call myself ...'. Hume has declared both explicitly and implicitly his basic assumption that selves exist and have agency, therefore acting to examine, introspectively, the content of mind. To perceive already presupposes a prior experiencing self.

Despite this weakness in Hume's approach, his scepticism of subjective experience as the basis for making judgements about the nature of mind or of perceptions, for that matter, stands. This bears restating in other words: the relationship between the component parts of a perception, of an object such as a red ball, for example, is not inherent in the object but rather is attributed to the object because of our experience of it. Thus, the actual relations between the disparate elements that make up the red ball may indeed be quite different from our perception of the object. This approach allows us to recognize that our experiences are fallible and that our subjective experiences are not immune from error, no matter how compelling or veridical they may be. This means we may not be able to expressly rely on our subjective experiences of what it is like to be human as the basis for our true knowledge of having a mind or what being a self entails.

Embodiment

So far, I have been looking at philosophical approaches to the nature of self and mind. More recently, there has been increasing interest in the notion of the embodied self, as exemplified in the writings of Raymond Gibbs in *Embodiment and Cognitive Science* (Gibbs Jr, 2005). He describes the embodiment premise as follows:

> People's subjective, felt experiences of their bodies in action provide some of the fundamental grounding for language and thought. Cognition is what occurs when the body engages the physical, cultural world and must be studied in terms of the dynamical interactions between people and the environment. Human language and thought emerge from the recurring

patterns of embodied activity that constrain ongoing intelligent behaviour. We must not assume cognition to be purely internal, symbolic, computational, and disembodied, but seek out the gross and detailed ways that language and thought are inextricably shaped by embodied action. (p. 11)

This approach prioritizes embodiment as the central element in the subjective experience of the self. It is noteworthy that embodiment is distinct from the body per se. Notions of the self are tightly linked to tactile-kinaesthetic activity, to recurring patterns of kinaesthetic and proprioceptive action. These are novel concepts that resist the temptation to separate mind from body. For example, perception is not something that only occurs through specific sensory organs in conjunction with particular brain areas but is a kinaesthetic activity that includes all aspects of the body in action. Gibbs, again, like Hume, is suspicious of the results of introspection in judging and determining the nature of the relationship between personhood and the body. So, the fact that, as individuals, we feel as if our bodies are mere receptacles for our thoughts, or vehicles for our beliefs, and ultimately that the self and the body are distinct and different does not make them so. For Gibbs, even if one's personhood may be more than the body, there is no self without a body.

The role of the concept of embodiment in creating a sense of self is often overlooked or understated. Yet in the psychopathological conditions that are the focus of this book, the uniqueness of the body in relation to personal identity is fragile and the place of the body in determining perceptual experience is strained. In particular, cases exist, for example in autoscopy, in which the unembodied self is experienced as the source of sensation and perception. This is a most curious possibility in the light of our generally understood reliance on sensory apparatus for perception.

Importance of the Empirical Literature

The scope of this book is the varying notions of the double in folklore, literature, cinema, psychopathology, and finally neuroscience. Ultimately, the aim is to come to a better understanding of the actual experiences that are present in the clinics with a view to examining what this means for our concepts of mind, self, and the embodied self. Often philosophical theories of mind rely on thought experiments, on imaginary cases. These imaginary cases almost always ignore what is known about the structure and function of the brain, have an erroneous understanding of the neurophysiology of the brain, or are plain impossible. I will be relying on the empirical literature, combining cases drawn from clinical psychopathology and the results of cognitive neuroscience experiments, to elucidate this most complex yet intriguing subject. To make the point clearer, Peter Unger (1990) in his book *Identity, Consciousness and Value* exemplifies the use of imaginary examples in exploring the nature of personal identity. His arguments are based solely on imaginary cases. He argues, for example, that there is a direct mathematical relationship between the coherence of a 'self' and the numerical composition of the brain, such that the gradual removal of cells from the brain and the associated question of how much of the person or the self is left. Essentially, he is arguing that the relationship between 'grain of sand' and 'a heap' is the same as that between 'neurone' and 'self'. This is a ludicrous position to take for all sorts of reasons but principally because it ignores everything we already know about the brain, namely that there are a variety of neural cells, structured in a complex anatomical but also functional manner, and finally that there are different functional sites. In short, not all neural cells are equal. Unger is aware of the risks attendant on his method: he says that when imaginary examples are 'part of a sensibly balanced methodology, a reliance on imaginative cases may be instructive' (p. 11). He adds, 'But, for true instruction to be gained, and as that methodical approach directs, the canvass of cases must proceed with caution' (p. 11). Nonetheless, he is not circumspect in his approach. He describes something that he terms 'spectrum of congenial decomposition' in which the gradual removal of water and cells occurs such that at some point, what remains is not a specified individual. His imaginary example appears to confirm for him that 'we are gradual beings' (p. 60), whatever that might mean. There is no empirical evidence that a gradual removal of any of the constituent parts of the brain will result in a gradually diminishing self. It is quite possible that there is a critical amount of a constituent part of the brain in a particular locus that has to be lost to result in a catastrophic event. Indeed, we already know that in Parkinson's disease, a loss of greater than 80% of the substantia nigra is needed to produce the features of Parkinson's disease. Thus, the mathematical relationship between the loss of material substance and the phenomenology of abnormal function is an empirical question. Sometimes it is linear, but this is not always the case. The relationship is not logical but empirical. Furthermore, the resulting impairment may have little to do with identity or the nature of self.

I have been arguing that fanciful examples are problematic, if not misleading, in exploring the nature of the self. The role of actual clinical examples in instructing our understanding is far preferable, in my view. Kathleen Wilkes in her book *Real People: Personal Identity without Thought Experiments* (Wilkes & Wilkes, 1988) makes the point: 'Personal identity has been the stamping ground for bizarre, entertaining, confusing and inconclusive thought experiments ... These alluring fictions have led discussions off on the wrong tracks; moreover, since they rely heavily on imagination and intuition, they lead to no solid or agreed conclusions, since intuitions vary and imaginations fail' (p. vii).

In essence, Wilkes is making the case that real-life examples are preferable to thought experiments that are unconstrained by the realities of the background conditions that determine what is or is not possible in the empirical world. Clinical cases are unusual and intriguing enough that we need not indulge in fanciful imaginary examples to clarify the nature of mind or self. I will no doubt return to these matters later. In short, the focus of this book is the role that clinical cases have in illuminating our understanding of the nature of the self and mind. The issues traverse terrain that overlaps with that of the philosophy of mind, but ultimately it is a book about psychopathology and not a philosophical treatise.

The Double in Clinical Psychopathology

Autoscopy and Its Variants

Doppelgänger refers to the existence of a double. There are at least two broad conceptualizations of the double in clinical psychopathology, namely experiential and ideational. Autoscopy is a term used to describe the experience of seeing one's body in a location outside of its expected position. There are six variants: the feeling of presence; autoscopic hallucination; heautoscopy proper; negative autoscopy; inner autoscopy; and out-of-the-body experience. So, it might be profitable to think of the variants of autoscopy as examples of experiential rather than ideational doppelgänger.

The term 'feeling of presence' describes a feeling of the physical presence of another person close to the patient who is not seen but appears to be just out of sight. The patient may, in addition, experience altered or anomalous phenomena regarding their body. Essentially, there may be a feeling of estrangement from the body – a feeling sometimes described as depersonalization.

Autoscopic hallucination involves the pure visual experience of seeing one's own body or its upper parts as if reflected in a mirror. In other words, in autoscopic hallucination, the perception is often, but not always, a mirror image of the patient. The hallucinatory experience is in natural colours and is usually of a motionless perception, or what is seen may imitate the gestures, movements, or facial expressions of the patient.

Heautoscopy proper also involves visualization of the double, but, in addition, there may be other anomalous experiences including a feeling of detachment, strangeness of one's body, as well as feelings of lightness and occasionally the experience of vertigo. The double may appear transparent, grey, or ghost-like. The double may imitate the patient's actions but may also act autonomously, not necessarily mirroring the patient's actions or movements. The characteristics of the double may differ from the patient's own body, such that it might be smaller or bigger, younger or older, and the gender may not be congruent with that of the patient. And surprisingly, the patient may feel that he/she can see the world through the eyes of the double. Some authorities regard the distinction between autoscopic hallucination and heautoscopy proper as superfluous.

Out-of-the-body experience involves seeing one's body from an outside perspective. The core of this experience is the separation of the body from the experiencing self. Typically, the body is observed from a detached and an elevated spatial position. The body is usually motionless during the observation. The surrounding environment is also seen from an elevated perspective. There is an associated strong emotional accompaniment and significance to the experience, and the emotions are more often positive except in cases where the experience is a precursor to an epileptic seizure.

INTRODUCTION

Negative heautoscopy refers to the failure to perceive one's own body in a mirror or when looked at directly. It is often accompanied by depersonalization and the loss of awareness of one's own body, sometimes termed aschematia. Negative heautoscopy can be unilateral, affecting only the perception of one half of the body. Finally, inner/internal heautoscopy refers to the experience of visual hallucination of one's own internal organs outside the body. Both negative and inner heautoscopy are rarely reported.

These phenomena are intriguing enough on their own merit, but they have the added cache of sitting within an age-old dispute within philosophy of mind and cognitive science, namely whether the self is separable from the body. In other words, whether autoscopy, heautoscopy proper, and out-of-the-body experience are clinical and concrete examples of the concept of Cartesian duality, thereby confirming the dual nature of the relationship between the self and the body. This issue points at the importance of autoscopy and related phenomena for illuminating the neural underpinning of the representation of the self. And whatever this neural underpinning might be, it will need to address the apparent facility for the 'self' to be separable from the 'body'

Delusional Misidentification Syndromes

There are other clinical conditions that are dependent on the idea of doppelgänger but not on the actual experience of the double. These conditions are distinct from autoscopy but depend on the implicit assumption that doubles of individuals exist in the world. These include the various forms of delusional misidentification syndromes: Capgras syndrome, Frégoli syndrome, syndrome of intermetamorphosis, syndrome of subjective doubles, delusion of inanimate doubles, and reduplicative paramnesia. These conditions are of great and continuing interest to psychiatrists, neuropsychologists, neuroscientists, and philosophers alike, because of their intriguing clinical presentations and the possibility of linking discrete beliefs to neural and neuropsychological underpinnings.

The Capgras syndrome is perhaps one of the best known and most discussed examples of the delusional misidentification syndromes. It is characterized by the firmly held but false belief that an impostor has replaced a familiar person. In Frégoli syndrome, the subject believes that an unfamiliar person is really a disguised familiar person, whereas in the syndrome of intermetamorphosis, the subject believes that the unfamiliar and familiar persons are identical because of shared physical characteristics such as hair colour or shape of nose. Sometimes, in the syndrome of intermetamorphosis, there is a dynamic aspect to the experience as rapid and inexplicable changes in identity are observed in real time. The syndrome of subjective doubles is characterized by the belief that a double of the self is abroad in the world acting in such a way as to damage the subject's reputation. Usually, the patient would have never met the double, but the existence of the double is presumed. The delusion of inanimate doubles refers to the belief that inanimate objects have been duplicated and replaced, whereas reduplicative paramnesia refers to the belief that places have been duplicated.

The concept of the double is important in popular culture and as a device in literature because of the implications regarding the fragility of identity by way of facial recognition and because of the challenges it posits to our notion of the physical uniqueness of persons, a uniqueness that is only truly put under strain in the case of identical twins. The possibility that persons, objects, places, and even time might not be unique is at the core of delusional misidentification syndromes. This idea that duplication is possible and even probable and that against better judgement it can be firmly held as self-evident and established even in the face of counterargument and factual impossibility raises a welter of queries, as much about normal processes as about abnormal phenomena. But the phenomenon also exploits extant, often implicit, beliefs in wider culture about the fact of doubles. Among the many questions is how we come to recognize faces, people, objects, places, and so on. And how we come to mark them as unique examples of a class even in the context of marked changes over time. I mean by this the fact that we continue to identify an individual from cradle to grave as the same person, despite significant changes in physical appearance over time. The urgent and continuing fascination with the delusional misidentification syndromes derives at least from the many theoretical, philosophical, and empirical matters that they raise. There is the added underlying assumption that these conditions may provide the basis for examining and investigating the neurological basis of delusions in general, but evidently also they provide the basis for examining the nature of identity, the features that determine the identification of persons, objects, and places – the distinction between identification and recognition. The uncanny feeling that is provoked when we come face-to-face with identical twins but that is not triggered when we are in the presence of a flock of birds, such as geese, or a garage full of the same make of cars in the same colour.

Finally, dissociative identity disorder (multiple personality disorder) raises the intriguing possibility that a single body may house more than one personality and that a duplication, triplication, or infinite multiplication of personality is possible. This possibility includes the notion that the personalities may be so distinct as to be unique identities, with unique biographies, preferences, and attitudes. This condition has entered the public domain and greatly influenced the notion of the double in fiction, and cinema. Even in its less pathological aspect, where there is an absence of distinct personalities, but merely contradictory aspects of self, this notion of the double is influential and is often used as a doppelgänger device, at least in cinema.

Summary

The concept of the double is well-established in human culture. This is evident in folklore and the various manifestations of this concept of the double, driven, as it possibly is, by the duplication of our physical parts and our presumed dual nature as matter, spirit, and embodied spirit. In the following chapter, I will explore the continuities and discontinuities in the concept of the double as it flows through from antiquity to the modern period.

CHAPTER 2

The Double in Antiquity

Do I contradict myself?
Very well then I contradict myself,
I am large, I contain multitudes

(Walt Whitman 1819–1892)

Euripides

Euripides (480–406 BC) was an Athenian tragedian who was born in Salamis and died in Macedonia (Figure 2.1). He is widely regarded as one of the three great tragedians of classical Athens, alongside Aeschylus and Sophocles. Although not as popular in his time as his contemporaries, Euripides is now recognized as a major figure in the development of drama and the arts. Euripides's life was closely associated with the political and cultural milieu of Athens. He witnessed the city's rise to prominence during the Golden Age of Athenian democracy and experienced the tumultuous times of the Peloponnesian War between Athens and Sparta. These events profoundly influenced his work and contributed to the development of his distinct dramatic style.

Euripides wrote around ninety-two plays, although only eighteen of them have survived intact. His works often explored complex human emotions, psychological depth, and the moral and political dilemmas faced by individuals in society. He was known for challenging traditional beliefs and highlighting issues such as the status of women, the futility of war, and the role of the gods. Euripides's plays often challenged societal norms and provoked controversy. Many of his characters were complex and multidimensional, displaying a range of emotions and motivations

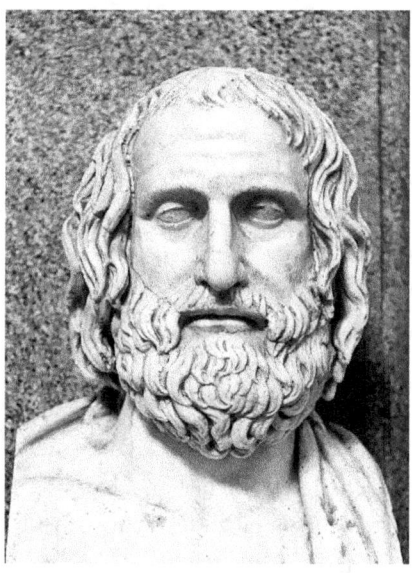

Figure 2.1 Euripides c. 480 BC–c. 406 BC (Public domain)

that were not always easy to categorize as purely good or evil. This nuanced approach to character development helped to humanize his protagonists and has been influential in the development of tragic drama in subsequent centuries. His plays include *Medea; The Bacchae; Helen;* and *The Women of Troy, Electra, Alcestis and Hippolytus*. In *Helen* (Euripides, 1954), Euripides deals with the central character in the Trojan Wars, Helen, reputed to be the most beautiful woman in the world, in her day. The standard tradition is that the goddess Hera promised Paris that Helen would be his, and under the guise of making a diplomatic overture, Paris seduced Helen and carried her off to Troy despite her being already married to Menelaus, King of Sparta. This abduction was the cause of the Trojan Wars. This play is an examination, albeit indirectly, of whether wars are worth fighting, and how far the said causes of war are real or mere chimera, illusions that drive actions.

In this play, Helen, who is thought to be in Troy, is represented as an illusion, a double. On the other hand, the real Helen in the mean time is in Egypt. Both Helens are physically identical and are simultaneously in different places. However, in the play's time and space, only one of the two Helens is seen by the audience. This is an example of an ideational double, a double that is not seen by the real person but is surmised to exist and understood to act outside of the province of the real person, and often in contrast to the desires and attitudes of the real person.

The True Helen Says

> And Zeus by his subsequent arrangements has added to my misfortune. He brought war upon Hellas and the unhappy Phrygians, to ease the swarming earth of her measureless burden of men and make Achilles famous among the fighters of Greece. The Helen who went to Phrygia as a prize for Troy to defend and the Greeks to fight for – that Helen was not I, only my name. Zeus did not forget me: I was taken by Hermes, wrapped in a cloud, borne through the secret places of the upper air, and set down here in the palace of Proteus, whom Zeus picked out as the most honourable of all men, so that I might preserve my chastity inviolate for Menelaus. (p. 136)

The proposition is that the true Helen is undeservedly the centre of these tragic events, the Trojan Wars, and is blamed with curses as the betrayer of her husband who brought upon Greece the pestilence of war. Earlier in the play, Helen had said: 'She [Hera] gave the royal son of Priam for his bride, not me, but a living image compounded of the ether in my likeness. Paris believes that he possesses me: what he holds is nothing but an airy delusion' (p. 136).

We have in Euripides's *Helen* the use of the double as a literary device to deal with a particular literary problem or to advance a viewpoint. The name Helen is associated with profound reputational damage, and in this play, Euripides seeks to limit the damage and to portray Helen in a different light. Helen says, 'My fair name is reviled for wrong I have not done' (p. 143). She goes on: 'In the first place, though I am innocent, my name is a byword of reproach; and if there is any worse fate than suffering for real crimes, it is suffering for crimes that were never committed' (p. 143).

Helen attributes her misfortune to her great beauty saying, 'partly because my very beauty led to my taking on an untrue and hideous appearance in the eyes of the world' (p. 143) and 'Beauty is a blessing to other women: it reduces me to this!' [contemplation of suicide] (p. 144).

The encounter of Helen and Menelaus is remarkable in that it both captures and sums up the incredulity and perplexity that attend the possibility that doubles exist. Menelaus had rescued the other Helen from Troy and was understandably astonished to find an identical other Helen in Proteus palace:

MENELAUS: Who are you? Whose face am I looking at?
HELEN: But who are *you*? We are both in the same perplexity.
MENELAUS: I never saw anyone more exactly like –
HELEN: O gods! Yes, there is something godlike in recognition!
...
MENELAUS: To me you appear to be exactly like Helen!
HELEN: To me you look like Menelaus! I don't know what to think. (p. 152)

In *Helen*, Euripides created a concrete poetic image of the illusory cause of war in the fake figure of Helen, a double of the true Helen. This theatrical double is closest to what Robert Rogers (1970) describes as a mirror image, a projected similar image that is not merely a similar self but an exact duplicate, but is yet not completely real in the sense of being corporally separate. Rogers cites the myth of Narcissus, who sees his face mirrored in a stream, as an example of this kind of double, the emphasis being on the mirror image being the focus of the myth of Narcissus. In *Helen*, the duplicate is corporally separate but constituted of ether, and disappears, vanishing into the air. In the myth of Narcissus, the double is created by the plausible mirroring effect of a stream. In Euripides's *Helen*, the duplication is a feat worthy of the intervention of the gods: Hera, Aphrodite, and Athene. Indeed, it is Hera who gave Paris for his bride, a living image of Helen compounded of ether. It could be argued that the use of the double in *Helen* does not attempt to be empirically true. It merely must be plausible to serve its theatrical purpose.

Plautus

Titus Maccius Plautus (c. 254–184 BC), commonly known as Plautus, was a renowned Roman playwright who is considered one of the greatest comedic playwrights of ancient Rome (Figure 2.2). Plautus was born in

DOPPELGÄNGER: ANALYSING 'DOUBLES'

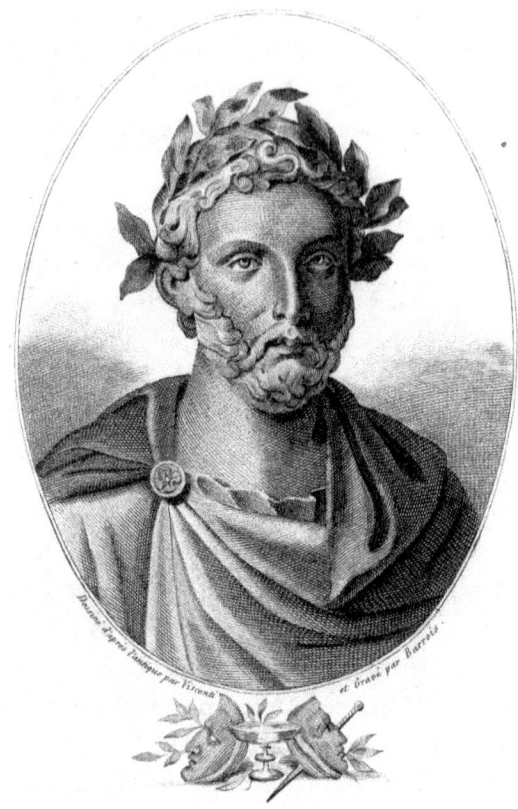

Figure 2.2 Titus Maccius Plautus c. 254–c. 184 BC (Public domain)

Sarsina, a small town in central Italy. Not much is known about his early life, but it is believed that he first became involved in the theatrical world as an actor. He eventually turned to writing and produced over 130 plays, although only 21 of them have survived in their entirety. Plautus's works are characterized by their lively humour, wordplay, and exaggerated situations. He drew inspiration from Greek New Comedy but adapted it to suit the tastes and cultural context of the Roman audience. His plays often featured stock characters, such as the cunning slave, the foolish old man, and the young lovers, who were put into comical and chaotic situations.

Plautus's comedies were known for their fast pace, witty dialogue, and physical humour. They often contained comedic elements such as slapstick, puns, and wordplay, which delighted audiences and made his plays accessible to a wide range of people. Though his works were popular among the Roman masses, they were not always embraced by the elite critics of the time.

While Plautus's works were highly successful during his lifetime, he faced criticism from some Roman intellectuals who viewed comedy as an inferior form of art compared to tragedy. Plautus's impact extended beyond the borders of the Roman Empire. His works were later translated and adapted throughout Europe during the Renaissance, and his comedic style influenced prominent playwrights like Molière and Shakespeare. The use of comedic devices such as mistaken identity, puns, and farcical situations can still be found in modern comedies.

In *Amphitryon*, Plautus has two doubles appear on stage: Jupiter (Jove) takes the form of Amphitryon, the leader of the Theban army, and Mercury takes the form of Sosia, Amphitryon's slave, for comic effect. This is a story of how Jupiter seduces Alcmena, Amphitryon's wife, by taking the physical form of Amphitryon. In the play it is Mercury's role to delay Amphitryon's return home by deceiving those who might interfere. He changes his appearance to look like Sosia, and the encounter with Sosia provides several comic opportunities. Alcmena has twin children: one is the son of Amphitryon, and the other Hercules is the son of Jupiter. At the end, when all the confusion is cleared up, Amphitryon is honoured to have shared his wife with a god.

Mercury tells the audience that his father Jove has taken a fancy to Alcmena and since he is bound to have whatever he fancies, Alcmena is already pregnant by him while at the same time carrying her husband's child. All this has come to pass while Jove is disguised as Amphitryon. And for Mercury to play his part, he too is transformed from Mercury to Sosia. In one of the encounters between Sosia and his double Mercury, Sosia says during the encounter:

> God help me, now that I look, he has my features-
> I've seen them in a mirror. We could be twins.
> My hat, my clothes – he's more like me than I am:
> Leg, foot, height, haircut, eyes, nose, even lips-
> Jaws, chin, beard, neck – no difference. I'm speechless.

> If his back's scarred he couldn't be more me.
>
> And yet I'm still the man I was:
>
> I know my master and my house: I'm sane . . . . *(Plautus, 1995, p. 25)*

Here is an example of a real identical double, both the true Sosia and his double are visually present at the same time, but the true Sosia experiences a sense of perplexity. Capgras syndrome was originally named *Illusion de Sosie*, after Sosia. This was apposite given that in Capgras syndrome, the patient asserts that even though the familiar other, for example, his father or mother, look exactly as they should, they have been replaced by impostors or doubles. There is genuine astonishment at the fact that a person who looks exactly as they ought to have been replaced by impostors. This astonishment is mirrored in Sosia's perplexed reaction in the play.

There is, in *Amphitryon*, the use of the twin motif that recurs in modern novels and films: Sosia remarks in the quotation above that 'we could be twins' and Alcmena is pregnant with twins, fathered by two different men. This reference to twins in *Amphitryon* forms the basis of another comedy by Plautus (2004), *The Brothers Menaechmus*. This play is often regarded as Plautus's greatest play. It is a farcical comedy that tells the story of two identical twins separated at birth, leading to a series of mistaken identities and hilarious encounters.

The comedic aspect is built on the mistaken identity of a set of twins: Menaechmus of Epidamnus and Menaechmus of Syracuse. In the prologue we learn that

> In Syracuse a merchant, it appears
>
> Begat twin sons, who from their earliest years
>
> Were so alike that neither nurse nor mother
>
> Could ever tell one baby from the other,
>
> So little was the difference between them. *(p. 103)*

The twins become separated after their father took one of the twins, Menaechmus, with him on a trip. Menaechmus is abducted and adopted by a merchant who lives in Epidamnus. The father dies and their grandfather changes the name of the other twin from Sosicles to Menaechmus. Sociscles goes in search of his brother and arrives in Epidamnus, not realizing that his brother lives there. Sosicles meets Cylindrus and Erotium, in turn, who appear to know him, much to his surprise. The situation becomes more absurd when Sosicles meets Menaechmus's wife and the consequences of the comedy of errors deepens to the degree that Sosicles is taken to be mad. But it is Menaechmus who is examined by the doctor for signs of madness and is pronounced insane, but this scene only reveals the fact that the doctor has little or no skill in determining whether someone is mad or not.

Menaechmus says:

> Whatever can have possessed those two to pronounce me insane? Me – who have never had a day's illness in my life! I'm not insane at all, nor am I looking for a fight or a quarrel with anybody. I'm just as sane as every other sane man I see; I know my friends when I see them, I talk to them normally. Then why are they trying to make out that I am insane – unless it's they who are insane? (p. 138)

The confrontation of Sosicles and Menaechmus was full of disbelief, surprise, and some anger. Sosicles's slave Messenio sums up the situation pithily: 'That man, sir is either an impostor – or your twin brother. I've never seen two men more alike; you and him – he and you – water is not more like water nor milk like milk than you two are' (p. 143).

The twin motif allows for a multiplicity of reactions, both people interacting with the twins who are unbeknownst to one another and of the twins themselves in responding to these reactions. So, there is the strange sense of not being recognized by someone who you know well, a kind of estrangement, and their disbelief at being recognized and responded to familiarly without any knowledge of the contexts and history being attributed to them. Finally, there is the uncanniness of being in the presence of an identical other, a feeling that strikes at the nature of the uniqueness of personal identity.

So, what is it to have an uncanny feeling, an unsettling feeling? In the context of encounters with identical twins, it is to be brought up against the possibility that our assumption of the uniqueness of individuals may after all not be true. It is impossible to both see and compare the identical twins at the same time. First, one must look at the one and then the next, and then second, compare both while holding the faces in mind. The ensuing astonishment and doubt of one's visual memory is the basis of the uncanny feeling. In *Amphitryon*, as in *The Brothers Menaechmus*, the doubles are unsettling not because of differences in character or personality, but merely by being physical doubles, doppelgängers. This uncanny experience refers to a sense of unease, discomfort, or strangeness that arises when we encounter something that appears familiar yet feels unsettling. It's often described as a combination of familiarity and unfamiliarity, creating a cognitive dissonance that can be quite eerie. In the context of the play, the uncanny feeling is triggered by seeing someone that closely resembles a known person but the known person is duplicated. The feeling is amplified because the situation challenges our expectations of what is normal or that is anticipated.

Romulus and Remus, the legendary founders of Rome, were twins. It is not exactly clear that they were identical twins, but there is nothing to say that they were not identical twins. The legend is that the twins were born in Alba Longa. Their mother, Rhea Silvia, was a vestal virgin, daughter of Numitor, a king who had been displaced by his brother Amulius. The twins are said to have been fathered by the god Mars. Amulius ordered that the twins be killed, and they were abandoned on the bank of the Tiber, left to die. The twins were saved by Tiberinus, Father of the River, and they survived with the assistance of others who cared for them at the site that was to become Rome. The twins were suckled by a she-wolf in a cave now known as the Lupercal. In a dispute as to which hill to build upon, Remus was killed either by Romulus himself or by his supporters. Romulus had preferred the Palatine Hill, while Remus preferred the Aventine Hill.

In this legend, we see how a mere difference of opinion between twins distinguishes between them and is the root of fratricide. We have then the possibility of psychological distinction even in the context of physical identity. Another way to understand this account is via the role of sibling rivalry as the source of tension between the twins, and potentially too, as the source of the need for differential traits or behaviours to distinguish between the brothers. In other words, even in the situation of physical identity, of doppelgänger, psychological difference seems imperative as a marker of difference.

The Epic of Gilgamesh

There is another tradition that includes the two protagonists in *The Epic of Gilgamesh* (George, 1999) as an example of doubles in literature. This poem probably dates back over 3,700 years ago, composed in Akkadian and passed down the generations. Originally thought to have been the work of Sîn-liqe-unninni, a scholar of Uruk, modern scholarship puts its origin in Babylon circa 1700 BC. The epic is about Gilgamesh and Enkidu. They are neither physically nor psychologically identical but are the prototype for the double act which is so prevalent in fiction, theatre, and films, including Holmes and Watson, Poirot and Hastings, and others. The first half of the epic narrates the story of Gilgamesh, the king of Uruk and Enkidu. Gilgamesh is described as

> Surpassing all other kings, heroic in stature,
> brave scion of Uruk, wild bull on the rampage!
> Going at the fore he was the vanguard,
> going at the rear, one his comrades could trust!
> ...
> Gilgamesh the tall, magnificent and terrible,
> who opened passes in the mountains,
> who dug wells on the slopes of the uplands,
> and crossed the ocean, the wild sea to the sunrise;
>
> who scoured the world ever searching for life,
> and reached through sheer force Uta-napishti the Distant;
> who restored the cult-centres destroyed by the Deluge,
> and set in place for the people the rites of the cosmos.
> Who is there can rival his kingly standing,
> and say like Gilgamesh, 'It is I am the king'?
> Gilgamesh was his name from the day he was born,
> Two-thirds of him god and one third human. *(p. 2)*

Despite his heroism, Gilgamesh was tyrannical. He harried the young men without cause, and took their brides, and at the same time despoiling the daughters of the warriors. And it is in the interest of curbing his excesses that the goddess Aruru created Enkidu:

> The goddess Aruru, she washed her hands,
> took a pinch of clay, threw it down in the wild.
> In the wild she created Enkidu, the hero,
> offspring of silence, knit strong by Ninurta.
>
> All his body is matted with hair,
> he bears long tresses like those of a woman:
> the hair of his head grows thickly as barley,
> he knows not a people, nor even a country.
>
> Coated in hair like the god of the animals,
> with the gazelles he grazes on grasses,
> *joining the throng* with the game at the waterhole,
> his heart *delighting* with the beasts in the water. *(p. 5)*

Enkidu was seduced by Shamhat, the harlot, and he lay with her for six days and seven nights, and thus was Enkidu's purity defiled and he was weakened, and he acquired knowledge and wide reasoning. He also lost his communion with animals. Enkidu left the wild for Uruk, where he challenged Gilgamesh:

> ...
>
> They seized each other at the door of the wedding house,
> in the street they joined combat, in the Square of the Land.
>
> The door-jambs shook, the wall did shudder,
> [in the street they joined combat, in the Square of the Land].
>
> ...
>
> Gilgamesh knelt, one foot on the ground,
> his anger subsided, he broke off from the fight. *(p. 16)*

The epic shows how two distinct individuals are drawn together, how they come to cooperate to accomplish joint heroic challenges, in this case, killing the ferocious Humbaba. But there is more to this story than the acts of two friends. Gilgamesh had a dream that his mother interpreted as follows:

> Mightiest in the land, strength he possesses,
> his strength is as mighty as a rock from the sky,
> Like a wife you'll love him, caress and embrace him,
> he will be mighty, and often will save you. *(p. 10)*

There is an intimacy that verges on the erotic in the relationship. Also, there is much emphasis on the physicality of the pair. Gilgamesh is 'fair in manhood, dignified in his bearing, graced with charm in his whole person' (p. 9) and Enkidu is 'like in build he is to Gilgamesh, tall in stature, proud as a battlement' (p. 13). This is a different kind of double; it gathers its strength by a doubling of the characteristics of the protagonists. The pair is equally matched and duplicated. There are subtle differences of personal traits and origins, but they could easily be non-identical twins. Where one is kingly, the other is from humble beginnings, indeed is closer to the wild and feral in us than the cultivated and cultured.

Rogers (1970) describes this kind of pairing as 'The Opposing Self' and references the relationship between Don Quixote and Sancho Panza as an example of this kind of double. In this reading of Don Quixote, Sancho Panza symbolizes the id, or appetitive nature of human beings, whereas Don Quixote is the ego ideal who imposes honourable duties and noble standards of conduct. Furthermore, Roberts introduces the role of psychic conflict between doubles of this kind and says that contrary to expectation, antagonism and dramatic conflict is the exception rather than the rule. In *The Epic of Gilgamesh*, there is physical conflict between the pair which is resolved by what Rogers calls 'perdurable empathy' between the protagonists.

So far, I have examined the role of identical doubles in literature, usually as a literary device for exploring the nature of identity itself either as the cause of momentous events such as war (see Euripdes's *Helen* above) or as a ruse for comic effect in Plautus's comedies. But I have also drawn attention to the non-identical double, a device of the use of one of the couples to act as a foil for the other, often employing difference as a means of amplifying the action or emotion resulting from tension between the couple.

Loki

Now I turn to a different kind of double, the kind that is exemplified in Frégoli syndrome. In Frégoli syndrome, the patient believes than an unfamiliar other is someone familiar and known to them. In other words, a total stranger is identified as a spouse or relative. In extreme cases, even the ethnicity of the misidentified person need not match with that of the known person. Cases have been reported in which an animal, for example, a cat, has been identified as a spouse or parent. The delusional belief underpinning this syndrome requires a belief in the possibility of shape-shifting, of the use of camouflage or disguise to achieve what is near practically impossible. It also requires the possibility of an individual being in two places at the same time – patients will say that they have no idea how the changes have been achieved but they are certain in their beliefs and hold an implacable conviction as to the veracity of their beliefs.

Frégoli syndrome was named after Leopoldo Frégoli (1867–1936), an Italian actor who was regarded as the greatest quick-change artist of his generation. He had the gift of impersonation and a remarkable ability to rapidly change roles from Wagner, through Rossini, to Verdi, for example. He played all over the world, including Brazil, Spain, Argentina, and the United States. He had a successful run in London, and he spent over a year at the Olympia theatre in Paris and returned several times until 1922.

Leopoldo Frégoli calls to mind Loki, a figure from Norse mythology, where he is known as a trickster god and a shape-shifter. He is one of the most complex and enigmatic characters in Norse mythology, and his actions often cause trouble for the other gods and heroes. Loki is depicted as a handsome and charming figure, but also as a troublemaker who enjoys causing chaos and mischief. He is the son of two giants, Farbauti and Laufey, and is often associated with fire, chaos, and transformation. In Norse mythology, he is responsible for many misdeeds, including the murder of the god Baldr, the theft of the apples of immortality, and the creation of the monstrous wolf Fenrir. Despite his mischievous nature, Loki is also depicted as a sympathetic figure, and his cunning and intelligence are often put to use to help the other gods.

Loki's character has been the subject of many myths, poems, and stories in Norse mythology. His complex nature and actions have inspired many interpretations and debates among scholars and enthusiasts of Norse mythology. In the *Prose Edda*, also known as the *Younger Edda*, a collection of Norse mythology and legends compiled in the thirteenth century by the Icelandic scholar Snorri Sturluson, there is an account of Loki, shape-shifting into a mare, and another of him changing into the likeness of a woman, in order to extract secret information that resulted in the death of Baldr. So, one could argue that Loki is a mythical equivalent of Leopoldo Frégoli.

There is much need to clarify how the term 'double' is used in literature as distinct from what pertains in psychopathology. In literature, Rogers argues that there is a distinction between manifest and latent doubles. In this approach, manifest doubles are very present and there is a physical similarity between the protagonist and the manifest double. In Rogers's view, this type of double has inherent limitations when deployed in literature as it lacks the necessary aesthetic distance that would allow the reader to identify with different aspects of the protagonist. In latent doubles, however, the different aspects of the protagonist are more subtly drawn. Rogers says:

> The elements of the psyche as they find expression in manifest and latent doubles are analogous to the state of the elements in mechanical mixtures and chemical compounds. Elements merely mixed together can be separated with relative ease, whereas those in a compound can be separated only by analysis, often with considerable difficulty. The elements which form the constituent parts of the compound may bear little resemblance in their pure states to the characteristics they have when combined. (p. 40)

Furthermore, Rogers argues that latent doubling allows for an uninhibited identification with the protagonist, permitting the reader to involve himself freely and deeply with the fortunes of a character. It is important to emphasize that Robert Rogers is writing from a psychoanalytic perspective and his preoccupation is with a psychoanalytic investigation of the double in literature. On the other hand, the goal of this book is to examine what the psychopathology of the double tells us of the neural underpinning of the subjective experience of the self. Examination of literature in this quest is to explore, insofar as it is possible, the continuities and discontinuities of the notion of the double from antiquity to the present, as exemplified in literature and in cinema. It is already clear that in clinical psychopathology the doubles are manifest but not always experienced. Sometimes the notion of the double is implicit and inferred on the grounds of experience, whereas at other times, the double is experienced, either felt as a presence or seen as in a visual hallucination. I term this distinction *ideational* double and *experiential* double, respectively.

Summary

In this chapter, I have drawn attention to Euripides's *Helen*, wherein Helen's double is an artifice to allow Euripides to examine the illusory nature of the causation of the Trojan War. This reminds us that in Greek and Greco-Roman theatre and in folklore, the use of doubles is as literary or dramatic devices to produce particular effects. In Plautus's comedies, the double serves a comedic purpose. In *The Epic of Gilgamesh*, the 'doubling' is, as Robert Rogers argues, a device to allow for decomposition of the potential characteristics of protagonists into component parts, a method that facilitates the possibility of the readers empathizing more deeply with the action of the literary work. In the following chapter, I will explore how the notion of the double is deployed in the modern novel.

CHAPTER 3

The Double as Other in the Novel

With an indescribable feeling of uneasiness he started looking around. But no one was there, nothing out of the ordinary had happened and ... meanwhile ... he felt that someone had been standing right beside him, just then, his elbows similarly propped on the railings.

(Dostoyevsky, *The Double*)

The concept of the double in literature is wide as it includes such disparate varieties as the actual experiencing of a version of the physical self, separate and apart from the self (the double as other), a belief that identical selves exist in the world but are only inferred rather than experienced, and the exhibition of distinct personalities in the one person (the double as duality). These varieties are unified by the idea that doubles are possible or indeed exist. At the outset, it is important to draw a distinction between notions of the double that underpin autoscopy and delusional misidentification syndromes (see Chapter 1), and concepts of what used to be termed multiple personality disorder and that is now referred to as dissociative identity disorder. The latter terms refer, at least in part, to the possibility that a single individual may harbour multiple identities. There is no suggestion that the multiple identities are doubles of the original identity, or that they are physically separable from the originating identity. There is no multiplicity of embodiment. In other words, these are not physical clones with independent identities. These conditions are interesting insofar as they contribute to our understanding of notions of individual identity, of individual psychology, and the possibility of the fractionation of identity into multiple, competing, and sometimes conflicting selves. Furthermore, there is a rich tradition in literature and cinema borrowing from Robert Louis Stevenson's (1850–1894) *The Strange Case of Dr Jekyll and Mr Hyde*, an exemplar of multiple personalities. I will deal, briefly, with this tradition later in the following chapter.

James Hogg's The Private Memoirs and Confessions of a Justified Sinner

In this chapter, I will focus on the novels that deal with the double motif as 'Other'. I mean by this, novels in which the double is a doppelgänger, a distinct other. James Hogg's *The Private Memoirs and Confessions of a Justified Sinner* (Hogg, 2010) is an example of novels of this kind. James Hogg (1770–1835) was a Scottish poet, novelist, and essayist (Figure 3.1). He was born in the Ettrick Forest area of the Scottish Borders, where he grew up as the son of a shepherd. Hogg was largely self-taught, but he developed a love of literature and began to write poetry and prose from an early age. Hogg was also a prolific poet and essayist, and his works often dealt with themes of nature, rural life, and Scottish folklore. Some of his most famous poems include 'The Queen's Wake' and 'Kilmeny'. Overall, Hogg is considered one of Scotland's greatest writers, and his work has had a lasting impact on Scottish literature and culture.

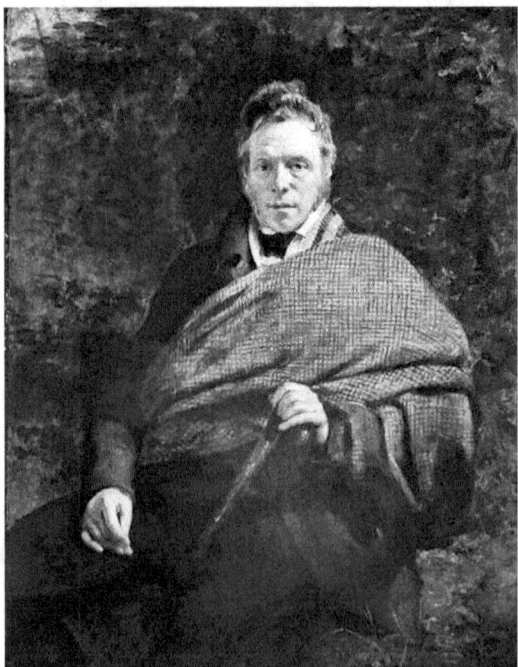

Figure 3.1 James Hogg 1770–1835 (Public domain)

He is best known for his novel *The Private Memoirs and Confessions of a Justified Sinner* (Hogg, 2010), which was published in 1824. The novel is a dark psychological tale about a man named Robert Wringhim who believes that he is predestined for salvation and can commit any sin without fear of punishment. The novel has been praised for its complex narrative structure, its exploration of themes such as religious fanaticism and psychological manipulation, and its use of Gothic elements. The protagonist Robert Wringhim's fanaticism leads him to be easily manipulated by a mysterious stranger named Gil-Martin, who convinces him that he has a divine mission to rid the world of sinners. Robert becomes increasingly isolated from society and begins to commit a series of murders, believing that they are justified by his faith. As the novel progresses, it becomes increasingly unclear whether Gil-Martin is a real person or a figment of Robert's imagination. The narrative also shifts between different perspectives and timelines, adding to the psychological complexity of the story. In the end, Robert is eventually brought to justice, but not before the novel raises questions about the nature of sin, faith, and the limits of human reason.

The book is in two parts: the first is the Editor's Narrative and the second is the Confessions of a Sinner. The theme of the double includes both manifest and latent doubles. The Editor's Narrative contains an explicit example of an encounter with a manifest double that produces consternation:

> Yet, mark me again; for all the things I have ever seen, this was the most singular. When I looked down at the two strangers, *one of them was extremely like Drummond.* So like was he, that there was not one item in dress, form feature, nor voice, by which I could distinguish the one from the other. I was certain it was not he, because I had seen the one going and the other approaching at the same time, and my impression at the moment was, that I looked upon some spirit, or demon, in his likeness. I felt a chillness creep all around my heart, my knees tottered, and, withdrawing my head from the open casement that lay in the dark shade, I said to the man who was with me, 'Good God, what is this!' (pp. 57–58, emphasis in the original)

The Editor's Narrative concludes with the consternation of two women having witnessed a true double of somebody who they had seen killed and who was very definitely dead. This incredulousness at seeing a double is a recurring theme in the texts I have so far examined. The experience calls forth the possibility that our visual sensory organ, the eye, is fallible, that our perceptions are subject to error, or that, indeed, our memory of faces and of the distinctness of a person may be faulty such that we come to misrecognize a stranger as a familiar other. The women say,

> 'It cannot be in nature, that is quite clear,' said Mrs. Logan; 'yet how it should be that I should *think* so – I who knew and nursed him from his infancy – there lies the paradox. As you said once before, we have nothing but our senses to depend on, and if you and I believe that we see a person, why, we do see him. Whose word, or whose reasoning can convince us against our senses? (p. 65, emphasis in the original)

This exchange goes to the heart of the perplexity that the idea of doubles induces, the induction of an atmosphere of the uncanny. Uncanny, in the sense of the twilight world of the instability and fragility of our perceptual world, of the degree to which our reason is dependent on the stability and certitude of the physical world and the durability and predictability of the world. We do not expect clonal doubles, and even in the context of identical twins, we still do a double take – we stop to reappraise our senses.

To be truthful, Hogg's account in the first half of his book of a manifest double does not mimic autoscopy, which is the closest psychopathological phenomenon there is, in any of its variants. What we have is a literary device, a narrative account that causes suspense and that provokes fear, dipping into the well spring of superstition to create a particular atmosphere, that of horror.

Hogg's approach differs from both later writers, such as Dostoyevsky's and Guy de Maupassant's, precisely because their accounts probably derive from personal experience and are drawn very closely to the factual and authentic form of autoscopy. For one, it is the protagonists in Dostoyevsky and Guy de Maupassant who experience the double and the sense of presence rather than that the double is visibly acting in the world in the presence of others who are in no way afflicted by disturbance of the mind.

In the second half of Hogg's *The Private Memoirs and Confessions of a Justified Sinner*, the doppelgänger is described from the first-person perspective, and here the similarity with Dostoyevsky's *The Double* could not be clearer:

> That stranger youth and I approached each other in silence, and slowly, with our eyes fixed on each other's eyes. We approached till not more than a yard intervened between us, and then stood still and gazed, measuring each other from head to foot. What was my astonishment, on perceiving that he was the same being as myself! The clothes were the same to the smallest item. The form was the same; the apparent age; the colour of the hair; the eyes; and, as recollection could serve me from viewing my own features in glass, the features too were the very same. I conceived at first, that I saw a vision, and that my guardian angel had appeared to me at this important era of my life; but this singular being read my thoughts in my looks, anticipating the very words that I was going to utter. (p. 89)

The astonishment and perplexity at the encounter with his doppelgänger are comprehensible and predictable given the strangeness of the situation, and indeed Robert Wringhim remarks,

> ...but as for his likeness to me, that was quite unaccountable. He was the same person in every respect, but yet he was not always so; for I observed several times, when we were speaking of certain divines and their tenets, that his face assumed something of the appearance of theirs; and it struck me, that by setting his features to the mould of other people's, he entered at once into their conceptions and feelings. (p. 91)

In this passage, James Hogg makes the comparison between the concept of the double, the replication of a unique single entity into its exact copy, a cloned copy, and that of Proteus. In Greek mythology, Proteus is a shape-shifting sea god who could assume any form he desired.

Proteus is also the name of a genus of unicellular, aquatic organisms called protozoa. These organisms are known for their ability to change shape and size dramatically, much like the mythical Proteus. The idea of a protean mechanism implies that the doppelgänger is independent of the original and that what it does is to mimic the original by taking its shape, shape-shifting, but also replicating its mental characteristics, although we need to be mindful that the doppelgänger may take on the opposite, diametrically opposite nature of the original.

Karl Miller (1987) defines the word 'duality' as meaning that there are two of something, and that it has also meant that some one thing or person is to be perceived as two. In this approach, the component parts may compete, repel, or resemble one another. But, implicit in the possibility of duality is the idea that both parts are true, that both Robert Wringhim and his doppelgänger are true. This is not the case with autoscopic hallucination, where the original perceives a simulacrum, but the simulacrum has no existence independent of the original. Furthermore, the simulacrum is not objectively present and cannot be perceived by third parties nor can it be authenticated by other sensory modalities outwith the visual. It is worth remarking that one of the senses of the term objective is that an object is liable to being perceived by more than one sensory modality. So, a visually perceived object can also be touched, heard, smelt, or at the very least observed by another person. This is merely to emphasize that the doppelgänger, in autoscopy, is not usually an object with the characteristics of objectivity. Karl Miller puts the function of duality in literature this way:

> Dualistic fictions, in all their dream-like generic idiosyncrasy, continue to impart experiences of duplication, division, dispersal, abeyance. Many are at once alibis and apologies. They are works which can find themselves both innocent and guilty. Hostile actions are ascribed to some further or to some foreign self, are performed by proxy – a performance in which scribes, in which fiction itself, are deeply implicated. The actions can therefore be said to be both admitted and denied. (p. 25)

In *The Private Memoirs and Confessions of a Justified Sinner*, Robert Wringhim can both commit murder as well as seek to shift the blame and guilt unto his doppelgänger. And the doppelgänger can both be a clone of Robert Wringhim as well as an independent entity who is protean in its manifestations. Robert Wringhim refers to the 'cameleon art of changing your appearance' and the doppelgänger responds,

> My countenance changes with my studies and sensations ... It is a natural peculiarity in me, over which I have not full control. If I contemplate

a man's features seriously, mine own gradually assume the very same appearance and character. And what is more, by contemplating a face minutely, I not only attain the same likeness, but, with the likeness, I attain the very same ideas as well as the same mode of arranging them, so that, you see, by looking at a person attentively, I by degrees assume his likeness, and by assuming his likeness I attain to the possession of his most secret thoughts. (Hogg, 2010, p. 95)

There is here a confluence of the physical and the mental such that in assuming the physical likeness, the doppelgänger also comes to know the inner psychological secrets of the assumed other. We begin here to glimpse the idea that the physical is an instantiation of the mental, and the gap between the physical and mental can be sealed over.

There is a clear description of the phenomenology of the double in *The Private Memoirs and Confessions of a Justified Sinner*, which requires James Hogg to at least have had personal access to real experience of autoscopy much in the same way that Fyodor Dostoyevsky and Guy de Maupassant had drawn on their own personal experiences in order to portray a veridical picture of what autoscopy is like. Robert Wringhim said of his experience:

I generally conceived of myself to be two people. When I lay in bed, I deemed there were two of us in it; when I sat up, I always beheld another person, and always in the same position from the place where I sat or stood, which was about three paces off me towards my left side. It mattered not how many or how few were present: this my second self was sure to be present in his place; and this occasioned a confusion in all my words and ideas that utterly astounded my friends, who all declared, that instead of being deranged in my intellect, they had never heard my conversation manifest so much energy or sublimity of conception; but for all that, over the singular delusion that I was two persons, my reasoning faculties had no power. The most perverse part of it was, that I rarely conceived *myself* to be any of the two persons. (p. 116, emphasis in the original)

What is notable in this detailed description of the phenomenology of autoscopy is the accuracy of the description of the topography of the double, namely, that it was always 'about three paces off me towards my left side'. In addition, Robert Wringhim makes the point that his sense of identity or his self was not intimately tied to either of the two persons; in other words, his conscious awareness was not explicitly or exclusively located in either person. It is of interest too that this experience of autoscopy is attributed to bewitchment, and perhaps it is unsurprising that such an unaccountable experience had to be attributed to magic or witchcraft. A natural science explanation was not yet available to the author at this time.

Robert Wringhim, the protagonist, is also presented to us as susceptible to mental malady. He is sometimes 'seized with a strange distemper' or is in a 'desponding state'. He has a multimodal visual and auditory verbal hallucination, in which,

> While I sat pondering on these things, I was involved in a veil of white misty vapour, and looking up to heaven, I was just about to ask direction from above, when I heard as it were a still small voice close by me, which uttered some words of derision and chiding. I looked intensely in the direction whence it seemed to come, and perceived a lady, robed in white, who hasted toward me. She regarded me with a severity of look and gesture that appalled me so much, I could not address her; but she waited not for that, but coming close to my side, said without stopping, 'Preposterous wretch! How dare you lift your eyes to heaven with such purposes in your heart? Escape homeward, and save your soul, or farewell for ever!' (p. 119)

In summary, James Hogg's *The Private Memoirs and Confessions of a Justified Sinner* is rich in its treatment of the concept of the double. Firstly, it explores the plural nature of the concept of the double as literary devices. Structurally, the book is in two halves, thereby already symbolically introducing the possibility of duality. We have two half-brothers, George Colwan, a generous hearted person, and Robert Wringhim, a troubled child who grows into a corrupt character who is a sinner and criminal. Both are born of the same mother and hence are half-brothers. Secondly, the book deals with autoscopy, in which an individual experiences either the presence of his double or sees the actual doppelgänger, an example of a manifest double with all the possibility of an uncanny atmosphere, potential for horror, and tense and thrilling episodes. There is much in the fiction that trades on the uncertainty of provenance and actuality of events in the way that the first half speaks to, colludes with, and collides with the second half. The effect is to shroud the narrative account in 'a white mist vapour', making rational judgement of the causes and veracity of events both problematic and unproductive.

Like the book, James Hogg is himself described by Karl Miller as 'a singular and unaccountable fellow – singular and plural in the romantic style' (p. 16). He was said to be illiterate in the sense that he could not read until the age of fifteen years and had no access to books beyond the Bible. Miller says that 'he was a peasant, whose wraith ... was once seen by an old woman' (p. 16), suggesting that, like Dostoyevsky and de Maupassant, the descriptions of autoscopy may have been based on real experience.

Hoffmann's The Devils Elixir

There is uncertainty about how far E. T. A. Hoffmann's novel *The Devil's Elixir* (Hoffmann, 2009) influenced James Hogg's *The Private Memoirs and Confessions of a Justified Sinner*. E. T. A. Hoffmann, born Ernst Theodor Wilhelm Hoffmann on 24 January 1776, in Königsberg, Prussia (now Kaliningrad, Russia), was a German Romantic author, composer, and artist (Figure 3.2). Hoffmann's life was marked by his deep love for the arts. Initially, he pursued a career in law, earning a doctorate and working as a legal advisor. However, his longing for artistic expression compelled him to follow his true passion. He abandoned law and embraced music, becoming a prolific composer during his early years.

Although Hoffmann composed numerous musical works, including symphonies, operas, and chamber music, it was his literary talent that brought him lasting fame. He is most renowned for his collection of tales in *Das schwarze Buch* (The Black Book) and his masterpiece *Die Serapionsbrüder* (*The Serapion Brethren*). These works display his flair for weaving elaborate and mysterious narratives, often delving into the supernatural and fantastic.

Hoffmann's stories were groundbreaking in their blending of fantasy, horror, and psychological elements. His imaginative storytelling

DOPPELGÄNGER: ANALYSING 'DOUBLES'

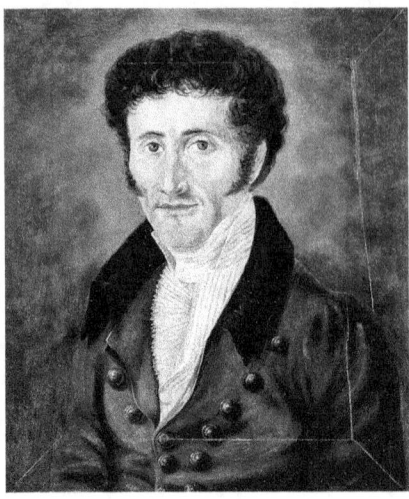

Figure 3.2 Ernst Theodor Wilhelm Hoffmann 1776–1822 (Public domain)

influenced and shaped the genres of Gothic literature and fantasy, providing inspiration to later authors such as Edgar Allan Poe and Nikolai Gogol. Apart from his literary pursuits, Hoffmann also excelled as a visual artist, creating intricate sketches and watercolour paintings. His artwork often portrayed scenes from his own stories, adding another dimension to his creative expression. He was also a composer, music critic, and jurist.

E. T. A. Hoffmann's life was tragically cut short when he died at the age of forty-six on 25 June 1822. Through his writings and compositions, Hoffmann left a mark on the Romantic movement and established him as one of the foremost figures of German Romanticism.

Hoffmann's novel, *The Devil's Elixir*, is a gothic novel, first published in 1815 and translated by an Edinburgh friend of James Hogg. Hogg's novel was first published in 1824 and deals with a similar terrain as E. T. A. Hoffmann's novel. *The Devil's Elixir* is, perhaps, the most influential of early Continental European dualist novels. The story follows the life of a young man named Francis Merdardus who is studying to become a monk in a Capuchin monastery in Spain.

The Devil's Elixir is a tale of mystery, suspense, and the battle between good and evil, and is considered one of Hoffmann's most important and influential works. The plot is complex, even at times confusing. There are numerous examples of doppelgänger. Earlier in the novel, Francis Medardus, the protagonist, sees the choirmaster's sister who we later learn to be Aurelia, and she is described as a most attractive woman in the full glory of her sex. 'She displayed above all a well-developed body of the purest contours, with the most beautiful arms and the most beautiful breasts, both in form and complexion, that one could imagine' (p. 17). Later Francis identifies this woman with Saint Rosalia whose portrait, at the moment of her martyrdom, hung at the altar of the chapel of his Capuchin monastery. Medardus is himself mistaken for Count Victor, and in this guise, he has a sexual relationship with Baroness Euphemia. In another encounter with a doppelgänger, Medardus sees himself: 'The door opened and a dark figure entered whom I recognised to my horror as my own self in Capuchin robes, with beard and tonsure. The figure came nearer and nearer my bed; I lay motionless, and every sound I tried to utter was stifled in the trance that gripped me' (p. 97). And Medardus recounts that 'I felt happy and relieved that the monk who was a horrible, distorted reflection on my own self had finally been removed . . .' (p. 109).

The number and appearances of doppelgängers are dizzying: a princess is identified with the Abbess, Francis Medardus is himself identified with his own father, and another unnamed monk is identified as Medardus, and Medardus himself has a doppelgänger who is described as a spectre. The most prominent example of a doppelgänger is of the character of Medardus, who is a doppelgänger for both Francis's father and for Francis himself.

There are examples of the mere sense of presence: 'As I hastened through the dark streets someone seemed to be running behind me . . . Looking round, I realised it was only the spectre of my double haunting my imagination, but I could not rid myself of it' (p. 175); autoscopic hallucination:

> I got up but hardly had I moved away when a man sprang out of the bushes and jumped on to my back, clinging to my neck. In vain I tried to shake him off. I threw myself on the ground, jammed my back against the trees, but all to no avail. He cackled and laughed mockingly. Then the moon broke brightly through the black pine-trees, and the pallid, hideous face of

the monk, the supposed Medardus, my double stared at me with its glassy eyes as it had done in the cart. (p. 194)

More unusually, there is an example of the doppelgänger's voice, an auditory verbal hallucination in the absence of any visual experience, which is recognized because of its characteristic stammer – 'The voice now sounded familiar to me; I had heard it somewhere before but not, I thought, so disjointed and stuttering. To my horror I almost seemed to recognise it as my own voice, and as if wanting to see whether it really was so, I imitated the stammer' (p. 154). All of these examples serve to create an atmosphere of uncertainty and disorientation, blurring the lines between reality and illusion and creating a sense of psychological unease. In his introduction to his translation of *The Devil's Elixir*, Ronald Taylor writes,

> ... Hoffmann's concern went beyond the spectacular presentation of a series of sensational events and coincidences. The course of Medardus's life is determined by the sins of his forebears. Ironically, he thinks that by ridding himself of the irksome restrictions of monastic life, he will find the freedom in which to indulge to the full the earthly desires welling up within him. Fate, however, has decreed other wise: to him has fallen the charge of redeeming the sins of his degenerate line, and after the vicious temptations and wanton brutalities have run their course, salvation finally comes with the transfiguration of his love for Aurelia in the moment of her death. This is the deepest meaning of Hoffmann's novel: Redemption through pure, transcendental Love. (p. viii)

There are some similarities and connections between James Hogg's *The Private Memoirs and Confessions of a Justified Sinner* and E. T. A. Hoffmann's *The Devil's Elixir*. Both works belong to the Gothic tradition and explore themes of supernatural, psychological, and moral ambiguity. They both feature protagonists who are struggling with internal conflicts and are drawn into dark and dangerous situations. In both works, there is a sense of duality and fragmentation, as characters grapple with multiple identities and conflicting desires. One of the most striking similarities between the two works is the use of the doppelgänger motif. In *The Private Memoirs and Confessions of a Justified Sinner*, the protagonist, Robert Wringhim, is haunted by a mysterious figure who seems to be a double of himself, leading him into acts of sin and violence. Similarly, in *The Devil's Elixir*, the character of Medardus serves as a doppelgänger for both Francis's father and Francis himself, representing their dark sides and leading them down a path of temptation and evil.

Both works also share a preoccupation with the nature of evil and the role of religion in confronting it. In *The Private Memoirs and Confessions of a Justified Sinner*, the protagonist grapples with the Calvinist doctrine of predestination, which he interprets as an excuse for his own sinful actions. Similarly, in *The Devil's Elixir*, the characters must confront the devil himself and make choices that will determine their moral and spiritual fate.

Overall, while there are some differences in tone and style between the two works, they both explore similar themes and share a common interest in the complexities of human nature and the struggle between good and evil.

Miller makes the further point that Hoffmann, more explicitly, influenced other writers including Dostoyevsky and Kafka. And that the doppelgänger motif came to stand for 'spells, powders, draughts, elixirs, wizard's wands and doppelgänger-sticks ... We were to enter a world – a world of spectacle and sleight – in which dramas of deception, detection, and pursuit of the double agent, would be an industry and a commerce' (Miller, 1987, p. 49). The doppelgänger motif continues to be influential.

Poe's William Wilson

Edgar Allan Poe (1809–1849) is one of the writers who inherited the mantle of the gothic and mystery genre from Hoffmann and Hogg. Edgar Allan Poe was an American writer and poet best known for his works of mystery and horror. Poe's writing style was characterized by its dark and atmospheric themes, exploring the realms of madness, death, and the macabre. Some of Poe's most famous works include *The Raven*, *The Tell-Tale Heart*, and *The Fall of the House of Usher*. He was a pioneer in the detective fiction genre with his stories featuring the fictional detective C. Auguste Dupin, which influenced subsequent mystery writers. Poe's tragic personal life was marked by financial struggles, the loss of his loved ones, and battles with alcoholism and depression. Despite his struggles during his lifetime, Edgar Allan Poe's contributions to literature have made him one of the most influential and celebrated figures in American literature.

William Wilson was written in 1839, just after Hoffmann's *The Devil's Elixir* and Hogg's *The Private Memoirs and Confessions of a Justified Sinner*, and is a tale of a narrator who encounters his doppelgänger while at school. The doppelgänger accompanies him throughout his life and is present at his death. This is a tale that explores the nature of conscience, in Freudian terms, the super ego, and that focuses on the conflict between good and evil. The narrator's doppelgänger is an exact copy of him and has the same name too:

> I had not then discovered the remarkable fact that we were of the same age; but I saw that we were of the same height, and I perceived that we were even singularly alike in general contour of person and outline of feature. I was galled, too, by the rumour touching a relationship, which had grown current in the upper forms. In a word, nothing could more seriously disturb me (although I scrupulously concealed such disturbance), than any allusion to a similarity of mind, person, or condition existing between us. (Poe, 2015, p. 728)

The similarity moved beyond mere physical similarity in physique to include dress, gait, demeanour, and speech:

> His cue, which was to perfect an imitation of myself, lay both in words and in actions; and most admirably did he play his part. My dress it was an easy matter to copy; my gait and general manner were, without difficulty, appropriated; in spite of his constitutional defect, even my voice did not escape him. My louder tones were, of course, unattempted, but then the key, it was identical; and his singular whisper, it grew the very echo of my own. How greatly this most exquisite portraiture harassed me, (for it could not justly be termed a caricature,) I will not now venture to describe. (p. 729)

At the end, only in death did the narrator come to recognize that his doppelgänger was indeed himself, and by stabbing him, he had stabbed himself:

> A large mirror, – so at first it seemed to me in my confusion – now stood where none had been perceptible before; and, as I stepped up to it in extremity of terror, mine own image, but with features all pale and dabbled in blood, advanced to meet me with a feeble and tottering gait. Thus it appeared, I say, but was not. It was my antagonist – it was Wilson, who then stood before me in the agonies of his dissolution. His mask and cloak lay, where he had thrown them, upon the floor. Not a thread in all his raiment – not a line in all the marked and singular lineaments of his face which was not, even in the most absolute identity, mine own! (pp. 744–745)

So, this is the doppelgänger as other, physically identical, and perceived as a physical entity outside of the self, but that is both distinct and not. In this case, the doppelgänger of William Wilson acts contrary to the self but, at the end, is discovered to be indistinguishable from the self. It is, perhaps, Poe's genius that while writing in the wake of E. T. A. Hoffmann and James Hogg, he was able to further extend the territory of the double motif, to re-imagine it as a separate self but intertwined, distinct but inseparable, contrary yet in union.

Dostoyevsky, Maupassant, Saramago, and Endo

It is the novels of Fyodor Dostoyevsky (1821–1881), Guy de Maupassant (1850–1893), José Saramago (1922–2010), and Shusaku Endo (1923–1996) that are most often recognized as being examples of fiction in which the double motif is central and constitutive. It could be argued that both Saramago and Endo, self-consciously, drew inspiration from Dostoyevsky's *The Double*. In this section, I will focus on these four writers, drawing out the commonalities and differences in the treatment of notions of the double from nineteenth-century Russian literature to contemporary Portuguese and Japanese literature. The aim is to use this as a platform for further exploration of how the concept of the double is dealt with by later writers such as Brett Eaton Ellis in *Lunar Park* and Stephen King in *The Dark Half*.

Fyodor Dostoyevsky (1821–1881) was a Russian novelist, essayist, and philosopher, widely regarded as one of the greatest literary figures in

Russian literature and world literature (Figure 3.3). He is known for his profound psychological insights, complex characters, and exploration of ethical and philosophical themes. Some of his most famous works include *Crime and Punishment, The Brothers Karamazov, Notes from Underground,* and *The Idiot.* His novels often delve into themes of morality, religion, politics, and the nature of the human condition.

Dostoyevsky's life was also marked by personal struggles and challenges. He was born into a poor family and suffered from epilepsy, which would continue to plague him throughout his life. He was also a gambler. He was sentenced to death by firing squad for his involvement in a political conspiracy, but his sentence was commuted at the last minute, and he was then sent to a Siberian labour camp instead. This experience deeply influenced his writing and political views. Overall, Dostoyevsky's contributions to literature and philosophy have had a lasting impact.

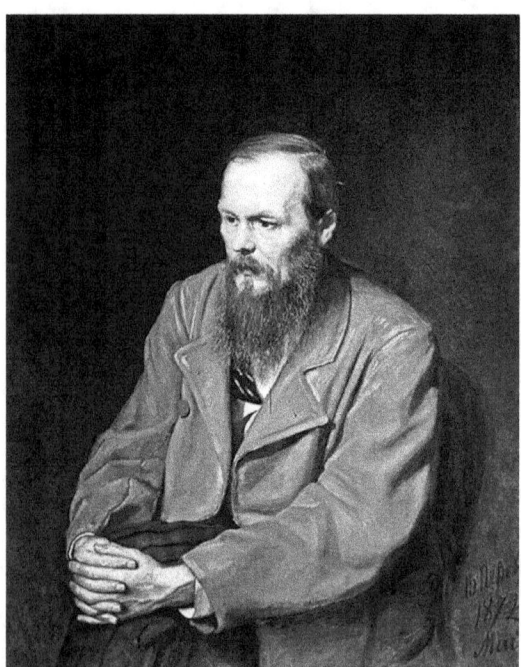

Figure 3.3 Fyodor Dostoyevsky 1821–1881 (Public domain)

In *The Double*, a novella first published in 1846, Dostoyevsky tells the story of Yakov Petrovich Golyadkin, a low-level government clerk who becomes increasingly disturbed after encountering his doppelgänger – an exact physical copy of himself who is more confident and successful in every way. As the story progresses, Golyadkin's mental state deteriorates. He becomes increasingly obsessed with the doppelgänger, who seems to be taking over his life. This is a story of the consequences of an encounter with one's own doppelgänger and predictably the results are tragic and morbid. The story ends on a bleak note, with Golyadkin being driven to a complete mental breakdown and a total loss of identity. The novella is widely regarded as a seminal work in the field of psychological literature, exploring themes of identity, alienation, and the fragility of the human psyche.

At the outset of Golyadkin's story, we learn that he is not mentally stable. He visits his doctor, Krestyan Ivanovich Rutenspitz, but the consultation seems to be at cross purposes as the doctor fails to fully comprehend Golyadkin's problems even though Golyadkin is trying his best to describe what his situation is. His demeanour is unusual:

> His grey eyes shone with a strange fire, his lips quivered and every muscle, every feature of his face twitched and shifted. He was shaking all over ... his lips trembled, his chin twitched and quite unexpectedly our hero burst into tears. Sobbing and nodding, beating his breast with his right hand whilst grasping the lapel of Krestyan Ivanovic's domestic attire with the other, he tried to speak, to offer some immediate explanation, but he was unable to utter one word. (Dostoyevsky, 1846, pp. 14–15)

Towards the end of the consultation, Golyadkin's expresses his persecutory beliefs. He says, 'I have enemies, Krestyan Ivanovich, I have vicious enemies who have vowed to ruin me ...' (p. 15). This is the prelude to the decline in his emotional welfare that led inexorably to his first experience of a sense of presence, a feature of autoscopy. In the immediate period before Golyadkin experiences a sense of presence, Dostoyevsky describes an identity crisis as follows: '...Mr Golyadkin now looked like a man wanting to hide, wanting to run away from himself. Yes! – that really was the case. Let us say more: now Mr Golyadkin not only wanted to escape from himself, but even hide from himself, to be utterly annihilated, to exist no more and to turn to dust' (p. 42).

Then we have his first experience of the sense of presence:

> All that is known is that at that moment Mr Golyadkin plumbed such depths of despair, was so tormented, harassed, exhausted, so bereft of any spark of fortitude, so disheartened, that he had forgotten everything... Suddenly... suddenly he shuddered all over and instinctively leapt a couple of steps sideways. With an indescribable feeling of uneasiness he started looking around. But no one was there, nothing out of the ordinary had happened and... meanwhile... meanwhile he felt that someone had been standing right beside him just then, his elbows similarly propped on the railings and – amazing to relate – had even said something to him, abruptly and hurriedly, not altogether intelligibly but about something very familiar to him and which concerned him. (p. 43)

Then the autoscopic encounter proper occurred in an impressive, remarkable description of self-recognition. Here was Golyadkin, initially knowing but yet not knowing who it was that he was seeing. Both a degree of familiarity but also a distancing from the facts. Indeed, an alienation from the self. 'The fact was, this stranger now seemed somehow familiar. That in itself wouldn't have mattered. But he recognised him – he almost completely recognised that man now. He had often seen that man at some time, quite recently even. Where could it have been? Could it have been yesterday?' (p. 46).

There then ensued a pursuit of the stranger along the streets, with Golyadkin becoming more and more agitated as he raced after the stranger. To his surprise, the stranger stopped right in front of the block where Golyadkin lived and then the stranger went up the staircase that led up to Golyadkin's flat, walking with the assurance of someone who knew his way, until he stopped right outside the doors to Golyadkin's door and knocked on it, and he was let in by Golyadkin's servant. Golyadkin followed him in.

> There was the stranger, sitting before him on his own bed, also wearing a hat and coat, faintly smiling, screwing up his eyes a little, and giving him a friendly nod. Mr Golyadkin wanted to cry out, but he was unable to; he wanted to protest in some way, but his strength failed him. His hair stood on end and he squatted where he was, insensible with horror. And besides,

he had good reason. My Golyadkin had fully recognised his nocturnal friend: his nocturnal friend was none other than himself, Mr Golyadkin in person – another Mr Golyadkin, but identical to him in every way – in brief, in all respects what is called his double .... (p. 49)

In Dostoyevsky's *The Double*, we have descriptions of sense of presence, possible autoscopic hallucination, and heautoscopy proper. To summarize these psychopathological states: 'feeling of presence' describes a feeling of the physical presence of another person, physically close to the patient who is not seen but appears to be just out of sight. The patient may, in addition, experience altered or anomalous phenomena regarding their body. Essentially, there may be a feeling of estrangement from the body. Autoscopic hallucination, on the other hand, involves the pure visual experience of seeing one's own body or its upper parts as if reflected in a mirror. In other words, in autoscopic hallucination, the perception is often, but not always, a mirror image of the patient. The hallucinatory experience is in natural colours and is usually of a motionless perception or what is seen may imitate the gestures, movements, or facial expressions of the patient. Heautoscopy proper involves visualization of the double, but, in addition, there may be other anomalous experiences including a feeling of detachment, strangeness of one's body, as well as feelings of lightness and occasionally the experience of vertigo. The double may appear transparent, grey, or ghost-like. The double may imitate the patient's actions but may also act autonomously, not necessarily mirroring the patient's actions or movements. The characteristics of the double may differ from the patients such that it might be smaller or bigger, younger, or older, and the gender may not be congruent with that of the patient. And surprisingly the patient may feel that he can see the world through the eyes of the double.

There is difficulty in determining whether Golyadkin's experiences amount to autoscopic hallucination or heautoscopy proper. Nonetheless, Dostoyevsky's description is remarkably accurate. In clinical psychopathology, the experiences are usually brief, temporary, and unsustained, whereas the literary example, here, is enduring and persistent. It is often said that Dostoyevsky modelled his characterization of Golyadkin on Gogol's Chichikov in *Dead Souls*, and that he also drew from Hoffmann's stories. The story and its relatively accurate description of real life autoscopy are rarely attributed to Dostoyevsky's personal history of epilepsy.

Dostoyevsky's first epileptic seizure occurred in 1839 when he was just seventeen years old. He continued to experience seizures throughout his life, sometimes several times a week. His epilepsy had a profound impact on his life and his writing, as he often wrote about characters who were similarly afflicted. Dostoyevsky's epilepsy also affected his personal life. He was often fearful of having a seizure in public and was embarrassed by his condition. This led him to isolate himself from others and to avoid social situations.

There is some debate among scholars about the exact nature of Dostoyevsky's epilepsy. Some have suggested that he may have had a form of temporal lobe epilepsy, which is characterized by seizures that originate in the temporal lobe of the brain and can cause hallucinations, religious experiences, and other unusual phenomena. However, there is no definitive evidence to support this theory, but there is no gainsaying the fact that he experienced convulsive seizures, whether or not they originated in the temporal lobes. Yet, Dostoyevsky's epilepsy remains a subject of interest and speculation among scholars and readers alike.

There are numerous references to Dostoyevsky's epilepsy in his letters (Dostoyevsky & MacAndrew, 1987). In a letter to his brother Mikhail on 9 March 1857, he wrote:

> On the way back (we came through Barnaul), I stopped in Barnaul at a good friend's. And there I had a stroke of misfortune. I quite unexpectedly had an epileptic fit that scared my wife to death and filled me with sadness and depression. The doctor (a learned and competent one) told me that, notwithstanding what other doctors had previously told me, I had *real epilepsy* and that I could expect to suffocate during one of the fits as a result of throat spasm, and that this is sure to be the cause of my death ... Judging by what I have been told by those who have witnessed my fits and seen what happens to my chest and my breathing, I should be certain to suffocate. (pp. 114–115)

In September 1857, Dostoyevsky had written to his sister Varvara:

> My sickness hasn't let up at all. On the contrary, the fits are becoming more frequent. Since last April I have had three fits while on guard duty and, on

> top of that, three or four others while I was asleep. They are always followed by weakness and sluggishness. It is very hard for me to bear ... the local doctors are powerless to help me. (p. 123)

Again, on 13 September 1858, Dostoyevsky writes to his brother Mikhail: My sickness is getting worse rather than better. Last month I had four fits, a thing that has never happened before, and I could hardly do any work. The fits are followed by a state of gloom and melancholy and I feel a completely broken man' (p. 137).

Dostoyevsky's epilepsy had profound adverse consequences for him quite aside from his descriptions of moodiness, depression, melancholia, and lethargy that were associated with the seizures. He wrote on 11 July 1878 to Yurev:

> The thing is that, for twenty-five years now, I have been suffering from epilepsy, which I contracted in Siberia. This illness has gradually deprived me of the ability to remember faces and events, to such an extent that I have (literally) even forgotten all the themes and details of my novels, and since some of them have never been reprinted since they were first published, I actually have no idea of what they are about. (p. 457)

We know that Dostoyevsky often drew on his own personal history of epilepsy in his fiction. For example, in the novel *The Idiot*, the protagonist of the novel, Prince Myshkin, has epilepsy and his seizures are an important element of the story. Myshkin's seizures are described as being both intense and debilitating. He experiences a loss of consciousness, convulsions, and sometimes falls to the ground. His seizures are also associated with a sense of euphoria and transcendence, which suggests that Dostoyevsky may have experienced ecstasy during his seizures.

One of the most memorable scenes in *The Idiot* occurs when Myshkin has a seizure during a dinner party. The other guests are horrified and unsure of what to do, while Myshkin's friends and family rush to his aid. This scene highlights the stigma and fear that were often associated with epilepsy in Dostoyevsky's time, as well as the deep bond that exists between Myshkin and his loved ones.

Overall, the portrayal of epilepsy in *The Idiot* is complex and nuanced, and it reflects Dostoyevsky's own experiences with the condition.

Through Myshkin's character, Dostoyevsky explores themes of mortality, suffering, and the search for meaning in life.

In The *Possessed* (Dostoyevsky, 2008), the protagonist Stavrogin experiences visual hallucinations and hints at experiencing a sense of presence:

> [H]e recounted that he was subject, especially at night, to hallucinations of a sort, that he sometimes saw or felt some sort of evil being beside him, mocking and 'rational', 'in various guises and with various personalities, but always one and the same, and I always get angry . . . .' These revelations were wild and incoherent, and actually did seem to be the product of a deranged mind. But even so, Nikolay Vsevolodovich spoke with such strange candour and such simple-heartedness, both absolutely uncharacteristic of him, that the former self seemed suddenly and unexpectedly to disappear completely. He was not at all ashamed to show fear as he spoke of his apparition. But all this was only momentary, and disappeared just as suddenly as it had come. (p. 756)

In *The Insulted and The Injured* (Dostoyevsky, 2018), Dostoyevsky's most overtly autobiographical novel, the protagonist talks about the degree to which his fictional characters take on a deep sense of reality that is akin to but not identical to autoscopic experience: '[W]hen I was living with my fancies, with the characters I had myself created, as though they were my family, as though they were real people; I loved them, I rejoiced and grieved with them, and sometimes shed genuine tears over my artless hero' (p. 29).

He also describes the vivid experience of seeing Smith, another character who had died, as if he were still alive:

> As it got darker my room seemed to grow larger and larger, as though the walls were retreating. I began to fancy that every night I should see Smith at once in every corner. He would sit and stare at me as he had at Adam Ivanitch, in the restaurant, and Azorka would lie at his feet. At that instant I had an adventure which made a great impression upon me. (p. 60)

He goes on:

> I must frankly admit, however, that, either owing to the derangement of my nerves, or my new impressions in my new lodgings, or my recent

melancholy, I gradually began at dusk to sink into that condition which is so common with me now at night in my illness, and which I call mysterious horror. It is a most oppressive, agonizing state of terror of something which I don't know how to define, and something passing all understanding and outside the natural order of things, which yet may take shape this very minute, as though in mockery of all the conclusions of reason, come to me and stand before me as an undeniable fact, hideous, horrible, and relentless. This fear usually becomes more and more acute, in spite of all the protests of reason, so much so that although the mind sometimes is of exceptional clarity at such moments, it loses all power of resistance. It is unheeded, it becomes useless, and this inward division intensifies the agony of suspense. It seems to me something like the anguish of people who are afraid of the dead. But in my distress the indefiniteness of the apprehension makes my suffering even more acute.

I remember I was standing with my back to the door and taking my hat from the table, when suddenly at that very instant the thought struck me that when I turned round I should inevitably see Smith: at first he would softly open the door, would stand in the doorway and look round the room, then looking down would come slowly towards me, would stand facing me, fix his lustreless eyes upon me and suddenly laugh in my face, a long, toothless, noiseless chuckle, and his whole body would shake with laughter and go on shaking a long time. The vision of all this suddenly formed an extraordinarily vivid and distinct picture in my mind, and at the same time I was suddenly seized by the fullest, the most absolute conviction that all this would infallibly, inevitably come to pass; that it was already happening, only I hadn't seen it because I was standing with my back to the door, and that just at that very instant perhaps the door was opening. I looked round quickly, and – the door actually was opening, softly, noiselessly, just as I had imagined it a minute before. I cried out. For a long time no one appeared, as though the door had opened of itself. All at once I saw in the doorway a strange figure, whose eyes, as far as I could make out in the dark, were scrutinizing me obstinately and intently. A shiver ran over all my limbs; to my intense horror I saw that it was a child, a little girl, and if it had been Smith himself he would not have frightened me perhaps so much as this strange and unexpected apparition of an unknown child in my room at such an hour, and at such a moment. (pp. 60–61)

In the event, the supposed apparition was a real perception of Elena, Smith's granddaughter, notwithstanding the fact that our protagonist had experienced repeated visual hallucinations of Smith. In *The Insulted and The Injured*, Dostoyevsky, once again, draws on his personal experience of epileptic seizures. He describes Elena's seizure as follows: 'And she flew at me, brandishing her fists. But at that instant we heard a piercing, inhuman shriek. I looked. Elena, who had been standing as though unconscious, uttering a strange, unnatural scream, fell with a thud on the ground, writhing in awful convulsions. Her face was working. She was in an epileptic fit' (p. 134).

Our protagonist, in this novel, is the authorial voice and has epileptic seizures, and this too is described but without the explicit features that he observed in Elena, just as we would expect in real life. He relied on the description given to him by Elena of what had happened:

> BUT as soon as I came in again I felt my head going round and fell down in the middle of the room. I remember nothing but Elena's shriek. She clasped her hands and flew to support me. That is the last moment that remains in my memory.... When I regained consciousness I found myself in bed. Elena told me later on that, with the help of the porter who came in with some eatables, she had carried me to the sofa. (p. 182)

To summarize, Dostoyevsky based his descriptions of seizures on his own experiences. One can speculate that he relied on his own experience of autoscopic hallucinations and of hallucinations in general for his fictional descriptions. This probably accounts for the authenticity of his descriptions.

What I have shown so far is that Dostoyevsky appears to have based his descriptions of seizures on his experiences and that as such it is also likely that he based his experiences of autoscopy on personal experience. It is important to emphasize that in *The Double*, Dostoyevsky does more than simply describe autoscopic experiences. In fact, even if the descriptions are based on his personal experiences, they depart from what one expects in autoscopy. The experiences are not brief, not transient, but sustained and enduring, to the degree that the autoscopic hallucinatory self is independent of the originating self and is able to interact with others and with the originating self. This is Dostoyevsky's genius – the ability to not merely depict an anomalous psychological experience but to exploit it for fiction, to turn it into a complex account that allows for the exploration of the nature of identity, of the nature of integrity of the self, and the possibility and potentialities of a clonal self in fiction.

Dostoyevsky captures, very well, the extent to which the double acts in malicious and malign ways to the detriment of the social reputation of the originating self. This is exemplified in the description, 'Good people ... never come in twos' (p. 98). The double usurps Mr Golyadkin's place with friends and with work colleagues. The double displaces him from their affection, from their regard, and ultimately drives him to insanity. The story ends with Mr Golyadkin seized by his doctor, Krestyan Ivanovic, and hauled into a carriage supposedly taking him to an asylum:

> My Golyadkin's heart was filled with a dull ache. The hot blood rushed into his head and throbbed; he was suffocating and wanted to unbutton his coat, to bare his chest and sprinkle it with snow and pour cold water over it. Finally he lapsed into unconsciousness .... When he came to he saw that the horses were bearing him along some unfamiliar road. To right and left loomed dark forests; all around it was bleak and deserted. Suddenly his heart stood still: two fiery eyes were peering at him out of the darkness and those two eyes were burning with malevolent, hellish glee. But it was not Krestyan Ivanovich! Who was it? Or *was* it him? It was! It was Krestyan Ivanovich – not the earlier one but a different, fearful Krestyan Ivanovich! (p. 163)

A novella that had started with an autoscopic double of the protagonist ends with the doubling of his doctor, the transformation of a benign doctor into a newly terrifying double. It is also an ending that mirrors Gogol's Diary of a Madman (Gogol, 1972), where the protagonist, following his descent into madness, is also transported to an asylum by carriage.

Guy de Maupassant (1850–1893) was a French writer, considered to be one of the greatest short story writers in the history of French literature (Figure 3.4). He was born in Normandy. Guy de Maupassant suffered from syphilis, which he contracted during his youth. Maupassant's health gradually deteriorated over the years. His later works often deal with themes of madness and mental illness, which some critics believe were influenced by his own experiences with neurosyphilis, a disease that

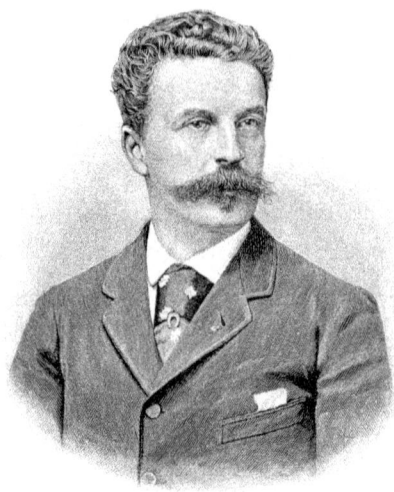

Figure 3.4 Guy de Maupassant. Nastasic/ DigitalVision Vectors/Getty Images

ultimately results in what was then termed general paralysis of the insane. Maupassant died at the age of forty-two, from complications of neurosyphilis.

In 'The Horla' (Maupassant, 2004), Guy de Maupassant deals with the subject of the double, including the sense of presence, autoscopic hallucination, and negative autoscopy. The story is presented by an unnamed narrator who gives an account of his illness to a distinguished group of psychiatrists and natural scientists at Doctor Marrande's clinic. The narrator lives on the banks of the Seine at Biessard, near Rouen. The narrator ends by describing a strange encounter he had with a ship, flying the flag of Brazil, while taking a walk along the Seine River and attributes his disease to this event. The narrator describes feeling a strange presence and becomes convinced that he is being watched by an invisible entity called the Horla. The Horla is a supernatural creature that feeds on human life force and drives its victims insane.

As the story progresses, the narrator's mental state deteriorates. He becomes obsessed with the Horla, believing that it is controlling his thoughts and actions. He begins to experience hallucinations and delusions, including the belief that the Horla has taken control of his body. The story ends with the narrator questioning whether the Horla is real or simply a figment of his imagination. He writes that he hopes his diary will serve as a warning to others who may be similarly afflicted.

So, this is a short story that deals with the same theme that Dostoyevsky explores in *The Double*. The title *Le Horla* ('The Horla') is a portmanteau French word made by combining the meaning of two other words. It is composed of *hors* (meaning outside) and *là* (meaning there). When translated into English, Horla is understood to be an outside presence or outsider and as such a title that speaks directly to the phenomenology of autoscopy.

The story is set in an asylum, with the protagonist telling his story to a gathering of psychiatrists and natural scientists invited by Dr Marrande, an eminent psychiatrist. So, we are swiftly introduced to the idea that his experiences are occurring, perhaps, in a psychiatric context. Indeed, the experiences, at their onset, include insomnia, hyperacusis, moodiness, and anger. Sleep was 'an absolute nothingness, a void, a total blank' (p. 237). He would wake, assaulted by an 'appalling sensation' (p. 237). He says:

> An unbearable weight was lying on my chest and another mouth was sucking the life out of me through my own. I would never forget the terrible shock of it! Just imagine a man asleep and in the process of being murdered. He wakes with the knife in his throat. He can hear his own death-rattle, feel his blood ooze out of him. He cannot breathe. He knows he is going to die but not why – that's exactly what it felt like! (pp. 237–238)

In Dostoyevsky's *The Double*, the protagonist is surprised, incredulous, and ultimately angry and suspicious when he encounters his double. In 'The Horla', the protagonist is terrified at the mysterious events that he experiences, that he endures. He named the invisible presence the Horla:

> Now. What should I call this ... Being? The Invisible One? No, that would not do. I decided to call it the Horla. Don't ask me why. So I was going to be stuck with this Horla indefinitely. Night and day I could feel it there. I knew it was close to me the whole time, yet totally elusive. I also knew for certain that with each passing hour, each passing minute, even, it was drawing the life out of me. I was driven to distraction by the fact that I could never see it.

> I lit every lamp in the house. Maybe given proper illumination it could be exposed. (p. 241)

The most unusual experience of our protagonist, and which is rarer still in clinical practice, is what is termed negative autoscopy. In this experience, a person fails to see their own reflection in a mirror:

> Believe it or not, though the room was bright as day, there was no sign of me in the mirror. It was empty, clear and full of light. But my reflection was not in it, despite the fact that I was standing directly in front of it. I looked at the large glass, clear now from top to bottom. I looked at it in terror. I dared not take a step forward, knowing that this being was in between. I knew that although it would slip away from me again, its own insensible body had absorbed my own reflection. I was so frightened! Then suddenly I saw myself begin to appear from the misty depths of the mirror, rising as if from a body of water. (p. 242)

This terrifying experience of negative autoscopy, intriguing and unbelievable as it sounds, is probably rooted on genuine experiences of Guy de Maupassant's. The actual nature of the experience is unclear, whether it is a form of agnosia, a deficit in visual perception sometimes termed object blindness, or whether it is a rare but recognized form of autoscopy described exactly as it is in the story. We know from his diaries and notes from 1891 onwards that he was undergoing rapid decline in both his physical and mental well-being. He wrote a letter to his friend and doctor, Dr Cazalis, in January 1891: 'I assure you that I am losing my mind. I am becoming mad. I spent yesterday evening at Princess Mathilde's, struggling for words, unable to speak, remembering nothing' (Lloyd, 2020, p. 30). By December 1891, he wrote, 'I am absolutely lost ... Death is imminent and I am mad' (p. 30). For a writer, a wordsmith, it was a deplorable, tragic end to lose the facility for words and of language. Maupassant cut his own throat during the night of 1–2 January 1892 but was saved. He lingered on for another eighteen months, declining into bouts of insomnia, manic pressure of speech, and epileptic seizures. He lapsed into coma for a few days before his death on 6 July 1893. We know that during the period of his mental decline, he complained that he had a doppelgänger on his tracks and he experienced hallucinations.

The Horla concludes with the psychiatrist, Dr Marrande, unsure of the nature of the experiences that had just been recounted: 'I am in as much of a quandary as you all. I cannot tell if this man is mad or whether we both are ... or whether ... man's successor is already in our midst ...' (p. 244).

José Saramago's (2005) *The Double* was first published in 2002. José Saramago was born on 16 November 1922, and died on 18 June 2010 (Figure 3.5). Saramago's life and works encompass a wide range of themes, including politics, social issues, philosophy, and human nature. Saramago grew up in a humble family and had a difficult childhood due to his family's economic struggles. However, he managed to pursue his passion for writing while working in various jobs. In the 1940s, he became a journalist, and his involvement in politics developed throughout his career. Although Saramago wrote numerous books, he gained worldwide recognition with his novel *Blindness* (1995). This thought-provoking work tells the story of a mysterious epidemic of blindness that spreads rapidly, leaving society in chaos. It explores themes of human vulnerability, societal breakdown, and the nature of power. Saramago received the Nobel Prize in Literature in 1998, which further solidified his literary reputation. His writing style was marked by long, flowing sentences without traditional punctuation, and he often questioned societal and political structures through his narratives.

The story of *The Double* follows the life of Tertuliano Máximo Afonso, a middle-aged history teacher who one day discovers that there is a man

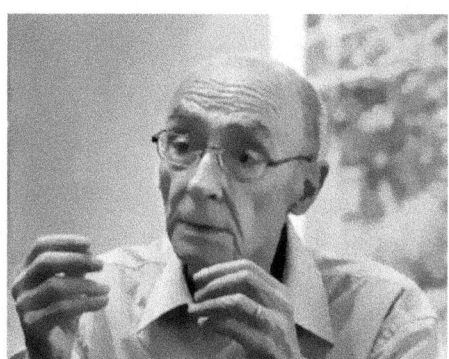

Figure 3.5 José Saramago 1922–2010. Presidencia de la Nación Argentina, CC BY 2.0

who looks exactly like him. The man is named Antonio Claro and is a minor actor in a low-budget movie. Initially intrigued and fascinated by this discovery, Tertuliano begins to investigate Antonio's life and ultimately becomes obsessed with him. As Tertuliano digs deeper into Antonio's life, he finds that he and Antonio share more than just physical similarities – they also have the same personality traits and mannerisms.

Tertuliano's obsession with Antonio becomes all-consuming, and he starts to lose touch with his own identity. He begins to neglect his job, his girlfriend, and his friends, and spends all his time tracking Antonio's movements and trying to figure out the meaning of their connection.

The Double is a thought-provoking and surreal exploration of identity, self-discovery, and the nature of reality.

The story is set in the context of Tertuliano's melancholia. At the very onset of the story, we learn of his depression: 'He is a history teacher at a secondary school . . . and is greatly in need of stimuli to distract him, he lives alone and gets bored, or, to speak with the clinical exactitude that the present day requires, he has succumbed to the temporary weakness of spirit ordinarily known as depression' (p. 1).

This is a novel that understands the features of autoscopy. Saramago describes Tertuliano's experience of a sense of presence. Tertuliano wakes suddenly and comes to the recognition that he is not alone, that there is someone else in his apartment. He gets out of bed in search of this other person, and as he searches '[t]he strength of another presence that had woken him grew slightly stronger' (p. 13) and as he moves into the corridor and approaches his living room, 'the invisible presence [grew] denser with each step'. But just as suddenly as the sense of presence had revealed itself, 'the presence like a soap bubble bursting, silently disappeared' (p. 14). The first encounter with his doppelgänger is itself unique. Tertuliano was watching a rented video film when he saw that a minor character, a hotel clerk, was his doppelgänger. He thought, 'It's me . . . and once more he felt the hairs on his body stand on end, what he was seeing wasn't true, it couldn't be' (pp. 14–15). We have here a similar consternation as in Dostoyevsky's *The Double*; the encounter is surprising but also alienating. To encounter oneself in another and in a strange situation is remarkable enough, but to do so, while watching a video film, with the detachment that the filmic visual image provides, produces a different level of alienation. It allows for microscopic examination of the physical characteristics of the other, and this is exactly what Tertuliano does. He carefully examines a frozen image of the hotel clerk, and rewinds the video to confirm what he has already concluded is a doppelgänger of himself. Except for a moustache that the hotel clerk sports, he is an exact copy of Tertuliano. As Tertuliano put it, 'it was not the effect of another impalpably, mysterious presence such as the one that had woken him, but of something concrete, not just concrete, but something that could be documented' (p. 16).

Saramago's *The Double* is not merely an opportunity to tell us a story but to explore what it might mean to have a double, to interrogate the concept of a double. Tertuliano says:

> [F]ive years ago I was the same as he was then, I mean both of us had moustaches, and more than that, the possibility, or, rather, the probability that five years on, that is, now, right now, at this precise hour in the morning, that sameness continues, as if a change in me would occasion the same change in him, or worse still, that one of us changes not because the other changes, but because any change is simultaneous, that's enough to send you stark staring mad . . . . (p. 18)

This is a notion of doppelgänger that we have not encountered before – a double that is not only a simulacrum but a physical identity that is co-dependent, and organically so. Any change in one is mirrored in the other. Furthermore, Saramago examines whether it is possible to change and yet be the same person. This goes to the very essence of identity; how is it possible that we might change either physically or mentally and yet remain the same person? What does it mean to be the same and yet be different? Further, Saramago has Tertuliano try on a disguise, wearing a beard, and then discovering:

> When he first saw his new physiognomy ... a terrible tremor inside him, the intimate, insistent, nervous palpitation in his solar plexus that he knows so well, however, this shock was caused not merely by seeing himself looking different, but, and this is much more interesting when we bear in mind the peculiar situation in which he has recently found himself, by his having a whole new sense of himself, as if, finally, he had

come face to face with his authentic identity. It was as if, by looking different, he had become more himself. (p. 147)

In speculating about what an actual encounter with his doppelgänger might be like, Saramago writes,

> Daniel Santa-Clara appears before you in the flesh, and the two of you stand there staring at each other just like two China dogs, each one a reflection of the other, except that this reflection, unlike the one in the mirror, will show the left side where the left side is and the right side where the right side is, how would you react if that happened. (p. 138)

This passage is quite crucial to understanding the physical relationship between the subject and his/her doppelgänger. Is the doppelgänger a mirror image or an exact replica? What is the spatial relation between the subject and the doppelgänger? Does the doppelgänger stand before the subject as in a mirror or is the doppelgänger standing alongside, sitting alongside, or lying alongside the subject? Finally, in out-of-the-body experiences, the observing self is often floating above the inert observed body, and does this spatial relationship have an understandable causal foundation? I will return to these matters later.

It is no coincidence that Saramago imagines a doppelgänger who is an actor with a minor role in a film and whose character is called Daniel Santa-Clara. The actor's own name is Antonio Claro. This raises the question of the relationship between a character in a film, Daniel Santa-Clara, and the real person behind the film character, Antonio Claro, who is the doppelgänger of our protagonist Tertuliano:

> [T]he first step on the road that will lead him to Antonio Claro, since Daniel Santa-Clara does not, strictly speaking, exist, he's a shadow, a puppet, a shifting shape that moves and talks inside a video cassette and returns to silence and immobility once the role he has been taught ends, while the other man, Antonio Claro, is real, concrete, as solid as Tertuliano Maximo Afonso, the History teacher who lives in this apartment and whose name can be found under A in the telephone book .... (p. 141)

Tertuliano makes a telephone call to the home of his doppelgänger Antonio Claro. The exchange between Tertuliano and Claro's wife is reminiscent of that between Sosicles and Menaechmus's wife in Plautus' *The Brothers Manaechmus*.

> Good afternoon, madam, but instead of responding in the reserved tone of someone addressing a stranger whose face she cannot even see, the woman said with a smile that shone through every word, if you're trying to fool me, don't bother, Excuse me, stammered Tertuliano Maximo Afonso, I just needed some information, What can a person who knows everything about the apartment he is phoning need to know, All I wanted to know is whether the actor Daniel Santa-Clara lives there, My dear sir, I will be sure to tell the actor Daniel Santa-Clara, when he gets in, that Antonio Claro phoned to ask if they both lived here. (p. 142)

As in Plautus' *The Brothers Manaechmus*, so in Saramago's *The Double*, doubles and doppelgängers provide the ground for much comedy. While in the Gothic novels of E. T. A. Hoffmann and James Hogg the doppelgänger is enrolled in deception, in mystery, in spectacle, here in Saramago's novel the doppelgänger allows not only a philosophical inquiry into the nature of identity, but there is also a return to the Greco-Roman model of comedy that relies on the double motif to play on notions of mistaken identity so as to create mayhem and absurd situations.

It is impossible not to wonder, when thinking about doubles, who the original is and who the copy, the duplicate, is. In autoscopy, this question can sometimes devolve to who the observing self is. Sometimes, the observing self is in the apparent virtual self, in the doppelgänger. This raises profound questions about the nature of the self, the role of the sensory organs in perception, and the possibility of a fracture between the physical material body and its sensory apparatus. These questions are not exactly what Saramago poses, but there is yet a true understanding of the problematic issue of the nature of precedence in the relationship between the subject and the duplicate:

> [T]he troubling question of who is the duplicate of whom, rejecting as improbable the hypothesis that both were born on the same day, but also at the same hour, at the same minute and the same fraction of a second, for this would imply that, as well as seeing the light at the very same moment,

they would at the very same moment, both have experienced crying for the first time too. (p. 157)

Saramago also imagines how Antonio Claro's wife feels about her husband's double – the possibility that an identical copy of her husband, with identical hands, would touch her, looking at her with the same eyes, kiss her with the same lips, and speak to her with the same voice, saying intimate and tender words. She regards this as a mad fantasy. This is an exploration of the uncanniness of the possibility of a duplicate of her husband existing and being indistinguishable from him. Here we confront the possibility that the uniqueness of each individual that we take so much for granted may be lost in some instances. And, of course, it is apparently lost in the case of identical twins.

The first encounter between Tertuliano and Antonio Claro is, as expected, pivotal to the story. Everything had led up to this moment just as it had done in Dostoyevsky's *The Double*:

> Tertuliano removed his beard and went in. That's what I call a sense of theatre, it puts me in mind of those people who like to burst into a room, shouting I'm here, as if their presence actually mattered, said Antonio Claro, while he emerged from the shadows and stood in the bright light coming in through the open door. They stood stock still, looking at each other. Slowly, as if painfully dragging itself up from the depths of the impossible, stupefaction wrote itself across Antonio Claro's face, not across Tertuliano Maximo Afonso's face, for he knew what he was going to find. I'm the person who phoned you, he said, I'm here so that you can see with your own eyes that I was not just having fun at your expense when I said we were identical. (pp. 193–194)

What this literary description does is to help us to understand the surprise, stupefaction even, that a person experiences when they are confronted with their doppelgänger in autoscopy. In the novel, towards the end, it becomes increasingly difficult to distinguish between reality and imagination. The complexities of identity are revealed when Antonio Claro dies in a car accident alongside Tertuliano's girlfriend and Tertuliano decides to take his place, which involves moving in with Antonio Claro's wife, Helena, and assuming the life of an actor, and so on. This shows that identity is more than just physical and psychological aspects but includes autobiographical memory, the intricate network of relationships and their influences, the varying roles, and the responsibilities that we have. In the end, even though Antonio Claro has died, while he is being buried, Tertuliano receives a phone call, and the story starts afresh – but this time, Tertuliano is Antonio Claro, and the caller is Tertuliano. The novel ends with Tertuliano taking a pistol and leaving the house. We assume that this is the prelude to suicide.

I have so far examined the novels of Dostoyevsky, Guy de Maupassant, James Hogg, E. T. A. Hoffmann, and Jose Saramago. These works have shown the variety of ways that the double motif is employed in fiction. I have suggested that the accuracy of the description of the nature of the double, regarding the degree to which it reflects the reality of autoscopy, may tell us something of the likelihood of the description being based on real-life experience. There is good reason to believe that Dostoyevsky, Guy de Maupassant, and James Hogg may all have had personal experience of autoscopy. The vivid and accurate descriptions are not by any means clinical descriptions but descriptions that are the foundation of storytelling. There is no slavish adherence to the facts of autoscopy, but merely an exploitation of the strangeness of autoscopy as the basis for fiction.

I want to now turn to Shusaku Endo's novel *Scandal* (Endō, 1988). Shusaku Endo (1923–1996) was a Japanese novelist whose works dealt with themes of religion, cultural clashes, and identity. He was born in Tokyo and raised as a Roman Catholic in a predominantly Buddhist society. Endo's novels often explored the complexities of faith and the challenges faced by individuals in maintaining their beliefs in the face of adversity. One of his most famous works, *Silence* (1966), tells the story of a Portuguese Jesuit missionary in seventeenth-century Japan who confronts persecution and religious oppression. This novel delves into the conflicts between Christianity and the traditional Japanese mindset, raising profound questions about personal conviction and spiritual struggle.

Endo's writings were deeply rooted in his own experiences and frequently examined the clash between western and eastern values, colonialism, and the incompatibility of different belief systems. While his works often focused on Christianity, they went beyond mere theological discourse to explore the human condition and the inner turmoil faced by individuals grappling with existential dilemmas. Endo was known for his profound introspection and was praised for his ability to create multi-dimensional characters. His writing style was often introspective and nuanced, probing into the moral and psychological complexities of his characters.

Scandal is set in post-Second World War Japan, and the story revolves around Suguro, a successful and famous writer. This is a complex novel and is often regarded as Endo's masterpiece. At its heart is the double motif, Suguro's doppelgänger, whose behaviour is the opposite of Suguro's. Suguro is a Japanese Roman Catholic, and in this he is like Endo himself, that rarity in Japanese society, a Christian. Suguro's earlier novels did not eschew the darker aspects of human life. While never avoiding the disturbing and the carnal, his earlier works instead focused on the tranquil and harmonious. Latterly, though, Suguro's novels found within the darkness and murkiness of his characters an opportunity for redemption. In other words, sin became the possibility of rebirth.

This novel, *Scandal*, allows Endo to examine not only unconscious processes and motivation, but also the hidden and secret recesses of the human mind. There is also in the novel an exploration of the degree to which a writer's inner life is affected by the plumbing of the depths and profundities of existence, such that in writing about jealousy or envy, the writer too is forced to submerge himself in jealousy and envy, and to become aware of the stench that is deep inside each person. And, to perhaps discover that he too is, if not tainted, definitely touched by the emotional material that he was excavating.

Suguro first caught sight of his doppelgänger at the reception for an award for his most recent novel. It was a fleeting sight, if that: 'Behind Kurimoto and this woman he saw another face. Suguro blinked. It was, indisputably, his own face. It wore an expression that could be taken either as a grin or a sneer. He blinked several times. There was no one standing behind the two editors' (p. 14). This was the beginning of a realization that he had a doppelgänger who was superficially different from him but whose behaviour revealed what is hidden, concealed even in Suguro, an upright and reliable person and a Christian too.

We come to know that Suguro's double acts within the liminal spaces of perverse eroticism, of sadomasochism, and even of murder. His behaviours are conducted in spaces designated for this purpose, such as 'love hotels', parlours where grown men dress as babies, out of the glare of publicity, so that a distinction can be kept between appearance and reality. To be mistaken for such a person was, of course, confusing for Suguro – 'You're confusing me with someone else. That wasn't me' (p. 17) – but this denial was met with disbelief and cynicism. So, this is a novel about appearances and reality, about the masks of ordinariness that people wear, and about the secretive life that expresses their true nature. Some of this is expressed through the ability of a painter to capture something of a person's true self, some vulgar aspect, that can be glimpsed in a facial expression or a look:

> It was a drawing of himself. In it he was staring straight ahead with a sneering smile on his face, the effect of which was that he been washed up from a realm of gloomy colours. While the face was certainly his, in the expression there was something, not exactly the vulgarity that Kurimoto had described, but something lewd and excessive. (p. 40)

Endo's use of the doppelgänger motif has some of the characteristic features of delusions of subjective doubles, a phenomenon that is a type of delusional misidentification syndrome. In delusion of subjective doubles, an individual holds an underlying delusional belief, a strongly held but erroneous belief that there is an impostor, a double who is identical in every way and is acting out in the world, in ways that will do damage to the individual's social reputation. The distinction between delusion of subjective doubles and autoscopy is that the double in delusion of subjective doubles is never observed but inferred from a primary belief that there is malice afoot of which the individual is the target. Technically speaking, this is a persecutory belief that is further sustained by the ancillary belief that an impostor exists who is responsible for the damage to social reputation. Whereas in autoscopy proper, there is a hallucinatory aspect to the experience and the double is usually seen, even if fleetingly. But this is rarely accompanied by persecutory accounts. In other words, the double is not usually perceived as the source of malevolent intent or action.

In *Scandal*, Endo explores the possibility that the doppelgänger can have an existence independent of the originating subject and can be observed by others: 'The strange thing is that it wasn't she herself who saw the ghost double, it was the girls she taught. While they were gathered in the sewing-room being instructed by their teacher, they looked outside the classroom window and saw someone who looked exactly like her standing in the flower garden. The whole class observed the apparition' (p. 140).

This idea of the materialization of the doppelgänger and the agency of the doppelgänger out with that of the originating subject allows the doppelgänger to function as a literary device, such as it does in Endo's *Scandal*, as it allows for action independent of the time and space of the originating subject, and hence there is far more potential for dramatic action and for mystery and horror. This possibility is exemplified when Kobari, a journalist who wishes to expose Suguro for his supposed hypocrisy, encounters the other Suguro:

> It was Suguro. But it was not the Suguro he had seen at the prizegiving, or the Suguro who had spewed out his oh-so-moral messages in the lecture-hall and on television. It was the Suguro whose face Motoko had captured in her portrait. As he walked past Kobari ignorant of his existence, his profile exuded arrogance and cunning and profligacy. (p. 164)

The conundrum for Endo is how to explain the mechanism for such an uncanny situation. This literary problem is never satisfactorily resolved. Suguro, himself, cannot be in two places at the same time. Yet, there is a suggestion that he has much more affinity with the doppelgänger than is easily explicable. For example, Suguro is invited to have a face-to-face meeting with his double, and when he arrives at the hotel, the meeting place,

> Oddly, he had the feeling he had seen this hotel before. He even had the sensation that he had been inside it. It was an inexplicable experience of *déjà vu*, like standing before a totally new landscape and having the impression that you had viewed the identical scene once in the distant past. But Suguro had no idea why he should have any memory of this hotel. (p. 206)

Saramago, in his novel, *The Double*, suggests that there is a symbiosis between the original and the double, affecting their physical and emotional lives. Whereas, in Endo's novel, no such explanation is forthcoming, and the reader is left with the task of determining how something so incomprehensible is possible. The encounter with the doppelgänger at his most perverse forced Suguro to acknowledge the 'filthiness' in himself, the baseness that he had been faintly aware of but not properly accepted prior to the encounter with his doppelgänger. Yet, this self-recognition did not involve an assimilation of one into the other. Suguro and his doppelgänger remained separate and distinct even in the moment of self-recognition.

At the end, Endo brings in the relationship between seeing one's doppelgänger and the imminence of one's death. This is a return to the idea of the *fetch* in Norse sagas, a premonitory event, presaging death. We have known from the outset that Suguro is dying from liver disease. It is never clear what the exact nature of the disease is or what the cause is, but we know that Suguro's condition is deteriorating. This link between the experience of one's doppelgänger and approaching death is treated by Endo as something to do with the ageing process:

> I read somewhere long ago that in our youth we live through our bodies; in our prime through our intellect; and in our old age we live through our minds as they prepare for the journey to the next life. And they say that the older we get, the more sensitive our minds grow to the shadows of that looming world. (p. 226)

The double motif in the novels of Dostoyevsky, Saramago, and Endo focuses on the double as a means of exploring, in their varying ways, notions of identity especially and sometimes of the possibility of hidden and secret aspects of the self. In the novels of E. T. A. Hoffmann and James Hogg, there is a way in which the double motif introduces the supernatural and inexplicable; hence, mystery and the metaphysical enter the discourse both as purveyors of action and as explanations for the inexplicable. It could be argued that this tradition is further developed in the works of Stephen King and Bret Easton Ellis in such novels as *The Dark Half* and *Lunar Park*, respectively.

Stephen King and Brett Eaton Ellis: The Double in Horror and Supernatural Fiction

Stephen King (1947–) is one of the most prolific authors of our time. He is primarily known for his works in the horror and supernatural fiction genres. King has published over sixty novels, numerous short stories, and several works under the pseudonym Richard Bachman. Some of his most famous and influential works include *The Shining, It, The Stand, Misery,* and *Pet Sematary,* among many others. These works often explore themes such as supernatural forces, psychological terror, and the dark underbelly of human nature. King's writing style is characterized by his vivid descriptions, realistic characters, and the ability to delve into the fears and anxieties of his readers. His stories often blend elements of horror, suspense, mystery, and psychological depth.

The Dark Half is a psychological horror novel published in 1989. It tells the story of Thad Beaumont, a successful author who is forced to confront his dark alter ego. The novel begins with Thad Beaumont, a college professor and a moderately successful author, who decides to put an end to his pseudonym, George Stark. George Stark is the author of violent and gritty crime novels that have garnered a devoted fan base. In a public ceremony, Thad 'buries' George Stark by revealing his identity to the world. However, soon after the burial, a series of gruesome murders occur in Thad's vicinity, bearing a striking resemblance to the crimes depicted in George Stark's novels. Thad becomes the prime suspect in the eyes of the police and the public, as his fingerprints are found at the crime scenes.

As the events unfold, it becomes apparent that George Stark is not merely a fictional creation but a physical manifestation of Thad's repressed dark side. Thad's wife, Liz, and their infant twin babies also become targets of Stark's malevolent actions. To save his family and regain control over his life, Thad confronts George Stark in a climactic showdown. The battle takes place in a surreal and nightmarish landscape known as the Castle Rock, a recurring location in King's novels.

The Dark Half explores various themes such as the duality of human nature, the creative process, and the concept of a writer's alter ego. It delves into the dark and sometimes unsettling aspects of an author's imagination and examines the consequences of suppressing one's darker impulses. Stephen King drew inspiration for *The Dark Half* from his own experiences with pseudonyms. Early in his career, King wrote several novels under the name Richard Bachman. When his true identity was revealed, he retired the pseudonym, similar to Thad Beaumont's actions in the novel.

The Dark Half received generally positive reviews from critics and readers. It is considered one of King's more personal and introspective works, blending elements of psychological horror, supernatural elements, and intense suspense. In 1993, a film adaptation of the novel was released, directed by George A. Romero, and starring Timothy Hutton as both Thad Beaumont and George Stark. While the film received mixed reviews, it retained the core concept of the novel and the exploration of identity and duality.

In *The Dark Half* (King, 1989), King takes the double motif and exploits it in a new and fresh manner. The double motif is illustrated by the materialization of George Stark, Thad Beaumont's pseudonym, when Thad Beaumont decides to stop writing under this pseudonym and to write in his own name. George Stark comes alive as Beaumont's doppelgänger. The novel is an account of Stark's serial murders as he moves closer to his aim, which is to kill Thad Beaumont. In this story, an imaginary character, George Stark, materializes and becomes independent of its originating agent and becomes autonomous and deadly in his intent and actions. As Thad Beaumont says, 'I don't have the slightest idea when he became a ... separate person. He seemed real to me when I was writing as him, but only in the way all the stories I write seem real to me when I'm writing them. Which is to say, I *take* them seriously but I don't believe in them ... except I do ... then ... ' (p. 189). As in Saramago's *The Double*, King examines the nature of the symbiosis between the original subject and his doppelgänger: '[H]ow can two different men share the same fingerprints and voiceprints and how can two different babies have exactly the same bruise ... especially when only one of the babies in question happened to bump her leg' (p. 241).

King continues, 'There was the case of identical twins who were separated by an entire continent – but when one broke his left leg, the other suffered excruciating pains in his own left leg without even knowing something had happened to his sib' (p. 241). But in the end, the explanation is typical of horror. There are preternatural forces at play, a confluence of unseen but evil entities lurking and waiting to enter material life and to enact malevolent effects.

Bret Easton Ellis's novel *Lunar Park* (Ellis, 2010) is another novel that exploits the double motif.

Bret Easton Ellis (1964–) is an American author known for his provocative and controversial novels. Ellis gained fame for his novel *Less Than Zero*, which was published when he was just twenty-one years old. This debut novel explored the nihilistic and hedonistic lifestyles of wealthy kids in Los Angeles and established Ellis as a voice of his generation. Ellis's works often depict a dark and disillusioned view of contemporary American society, dealing with themes such as alienation, consumerism, and the moral decay of modern culture. He is known for his unflinching portrayal of violence, sex, and drug use, challenging societal norms, and exploring the darker aspects of human nature.

Lunar Park, published in 2005, marked a departure from Ellis's previous works. It is a metafictional novel blending elements of horror, autobiography, and psychological thriller. The story follows a fictionalized version of Ellis himself, as he navigates the disturbing events that follow the release of his most famous novel, *American Psycho*. *Lunar Park* is an introspective work that explores themes of identity, fatherhood, and haunted pasts.

Lunar Park is written as an autobiography of Ellis, the writer, such that it merges facts and fancy, making it impossible to distinguish between reality and fiction. In taking this approach, it gives credence to the impossible while at the same time forcing the reader to suspend judgement and disbelief.

The novel is narrated by a fictionalized version of Bret Easton Ellis, who shares many similarities with the real-life author. The story begins with Ellis living a seemingly idyllic life in the suburbs with his wife Jayne Dennis and their son Robby. However, their domestic tranquillity is shattered when a series of bizarre and unsettling events occur. A mysterious presence known as 'the writer' begins tormenting Ellis, leading him to question his sanity and the nature of reality. As the narrative unfolds, Ellis delves into his own troubled past and confronts the demons that have haunted him throughout his life. He reflects on his tumultuous relationships, drug addiction, and the impact of his controversial novels on both him and society.

Lunar Park draws inspiration from classic Gothic literature and psychological thrillers. The fictional Ellis becomes entangled in a ghostly mystery surrounding the murder of a young boy named Jeremy, whose death seems connected to Ellis's past. The boundaries between fiction and reality blur further as the novel begins to mirror Ellis's own works, including *American Psycho* and *Less Than Zero*. The novel also examines the nature of fame and the impact of a writer's work on their personal life. It delves into the darker aspects of human nature, exploring the blurred lines between good and evil, and sanity and madness.

There are references to sense of presence, to autoscopy proper, and to other forms of abnormal experiences that rely on notions of the double but that are distinct from autoscopy. These are reduplicative paramnesia, a condition in which a person believes that a place has been duplicated such that two places exist that are identical in every way yet are distinct. There is also an example of auto-Frégoli syndrome, a state in which an individual believes that his own physical facial characteristics have been altered such that he no longer looks like himself but nonetheless he is still psychologically the same person.

But, perhaps the most compelling account is that of the 'writer', who is the alter ego of Ellis – a detached ego, distinct from Ellis, who writes his novels. This is a powerful idea, one that suggests that a self-monitoring awareness exists, a consciousness of one's actions but as if it were from outside. This experience is often described in depersonalization, where a sense of estrangement from one's own actions and perceptions occurs. Usually, this is a profoundly distressing experience that is difficult to describe but that entails a distancing from the self, an alienation that renders consciousness burdensome because it envelopes every action and perception with a distinctly unpleasant and disabling numbness.

Jorge Luis Borges's account in his short description 'Borges and I' (Borges, 1964) deals with this phenomenon. Borges writes,

> The other one, the one called Borges, is the one things happen to. I walk through the streets of Buenos Aires and stop for a moment, perhaps mechanically now, to look at the arch of an entrance hall and the grillwork on the gate; I know of Borges from the mail and see his name on the list of professors or in a biographical dictionary. (p. 282)

This experience speaks to the possibility of an observing self that is disconnected from action, that ponders and observes, but that is not integrated with the agentic self. And as in Ellis and Borges, there is a struggle, sometimes a conflict, between these two aspects of self. Borges puts it like this: 'Years ago I tried to free myself from him and went from the mythologies of the suburbs to the games with time and infinity, but those games belong to Borges now and I shall have to imagine other things. Thus my life is a flight and I lose everything and everything belongs to oblivion, or to him' (pp. 282–283).

There is here in Borges a sadness of tone, even a regret that the agency of the writer and the preoccupation of the writer are distinct and contradictory to his own needs and predilections. Borges develops this theme even further in 'The Other' (Borges, 1977), an account of an encounter with his doppelgänger. It was a horrifying experience followed by sleepless nights. The experience occurred in the setting of fatigue and was preceded by déjà vu and then a realization that a man had joined him on a bench, sitting facing the Charles River in Cambridge. The exchange between them is intriguing:

> 'Sir,' I said, turning to the other man, 'are you an Uruguayan or an Argentine?'
> Argentine, but I've lived in Geneva since 1914,' he replied.
> There was a long silence. 'At number seventeen Malagnou – across from the Orthodox church?' I asked.
> He answered in the affirmative,
> 'In that case,' I said straight out, 'your name is Jorge Luis Borges. I, too, am Jorge Luis Borges. This is 1969 and we're in the city of Cambridge.'
> (p. 4)

There then ensues anecdotes and reminiscences, some shared and others not, and talk of literature, and discussion of Dostoyevsky, including Dostoyevsky's *The Double*. As for the explanation of the encounter, Borges opts for dreaming, but who exactly was dreaming the other was left unresolved.

Summary

In this chapter, I have examined the treatment of the double motif, principally in the novels of Dostoyevsky, James Hogg, José Saramago, and Shusaku Endo. I have shown the continuities and discontinuities over time and over cultural space. In addition, I have highlighted the fact that writers with likely personal experience of autoscopy write with a degree of fidelity to the actuality of autoscopy but nonetheless exploit the reality of the experience to serve a fictional purpose. What is plain is that the double motif allows for an exploration of the nature of personal identity – whether physical identity is the repository of identity and how far psychological identity is instantiated in the physical. Saramago's *The Double* examines these matters in detail and shows that physical identity does not determine psychological identity. Indeed, autobiographical memory is predicated on time and place, irrespective of physical identity. This conclusion is already evident in the lives of identical twins.

In addition, the double motif allows for the different aspects of the inner lives of individuals to be explored. So, the dark and hidden aspects of a superficially integrated and harmonious life can be examined and can be split off and materialized in a physically identical other. Lastly, in the novels of King, Ellis, and Borges, we see the possibility of an individual, writing in the first person, encountering aspects of the self, who baffles, challenges, battles with, and ultimately seeks to destroy the originating self. While these accounts are compelling and intriguing, they are distinct from and quite unlike what it is like to experience autoscopy – distinct in the sense that in autoscopy, the embodied other is temporary, transient, and dependent on the originating self for sustenance and existence. The fictional doppelgänger takes a variety of forms determined by the inner logic of the narrative, and as such is not limited by the structure of the neurologically determined phenomena.

In the following chapter, I will examine the portrayal of the double as duality in fiction. In this conceptualization of the double, there is no corporeal other, visually manifest, and distinct. The double is part of the person, but exhibits different aspects of the self, often contradictory and perverse, warring, and unintegrated aspects of the self.

CHAPTER 4

The Double as Duality in Fiction

Although I had now two characters as well as two appearances, one was wholly evil, and the other was still the old Henry Jekyll, that incongruous compound of whose reformation and improvement I had already learned to despair.

(Robert Louis Stevenson 1850–1894)

In fiction, the notion of duality refers to the presence of contrasting or opposing elements within a story. It often involves the representation of two opposing forces, themes, or characters that complement and highlight each other. This duality is commonly used to explore various concepts such as good versus evil, light versus darkness, order versus chaos, or even the complexity of human nature. By presenting these opposing forces, writers create tension, depth, and complexity within their narratives, ultimately allowing readers to engage with conflicting ideas and perspectives. Duality in fiction can add richness to the story, and can enable deeper exploration of, for example, the nature of identity, the contrasting meanings of good and evil, and what guilt and personal responsibility stand for. In this chapter, I will be examining how the double motif takes the form of duality, and how this differs from the manner in which the double motif is represented as an embodied other.

Robert Louis Stevenson's The Strange Case of Dr Jekyll and Mr Hyde

Robert Louis Stevenson (1850–1894) was born in Edinburgh (Figure 4.1). He was a novelist, poet, and travel writer. His works spanned various genres, including adventure, horror, and historical fiction. *The Strange Case of Dr Jekyll and Mr Hyde* was published in 1886 and explores the duality

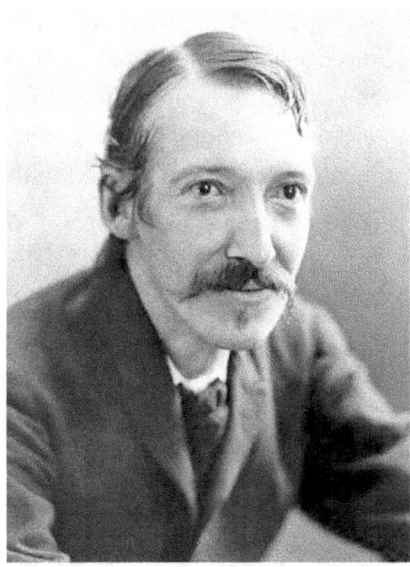

Figure 4.1 Robert Louis Stevenson 1850–1894 (Public domain)

of human nature. The tale follows the respected Dr Henry Jekyll, who conducts a dangerous experiment to separate his good and evil selves. Jekyll's experiment sets Mr Hyde, a depraved alter ego, free to indulge in his illicit and dark desires. As the story unfolds, Jekyll's attempts to control Hyde become futile, leading to unwanted consequences.

Beyond this iconic novella, Stevenson's repertoire includes other notable works such as *Treasure Island* and *Kidnapped*. Stevenson's writings often focused on themes of identity, morality, and the consequences of one's actions. In addition to his fiction, Stevenson's travel writings include *Travels with a Donkey in the Cevennes* and *In the South Seas*.

In *Dr Jekyll and Mr Hyde* (Stevenson & Middleton, 1993), Stevenson describes Mr Hyde as 'There is something wrong with his appearance; something displeasing, something downright detestable. I never saw a man I so disliked, and yet I scarce know why. He must be deformed somewhere; he gives a strong feeling of deformity, although I couldn't specify the point' (p. 7). Dr Jekyll, on the other hand, is described as 'a large, well-made, smooth-faced man of fifty, with something of a slyish cast perhaps, but every mark of capacity and kindness' (p. 14). These are the two aspects of the same person: Jekyll is the genial and respectable doctor, and Hyde is the alter ego, who is described as pure evil. In this account of the double as duality, the difference between the two aspects is manifest as much in physique as in psychology. But not simply that these aspects are distinct but that good and evil and psychology and morality have an influence that is discernible in physiognomy. Good is manifestly genial, whereas evil is grotesque.

When we finally come to a realization that both Dr Jekyll and Mr Hyde are one and the same person, we witness by proxy the transformation of one to the other as follows:

> He put the glass to his lips, and drank at one gulp. A cry followed; he reeled, staggered, clutched at the table and held on, staring with injected eyes, gasping with open mouth; and as I looked, there came, I thought, a change – he seemed to swell – his face became suddenly black, and the features seemed to melt and alter – and the next moment I had sprung to my feet and leaped against the wall, my arm raised to shield me from that prodigy, my mind submerged in terror.
>
> 'O God!' I screamed, and 'O God!' again and again; for there before my eyes – pale and shaken, and half fainting, and groping before him with his hands, like a man restored from death – there stood Henry Jekyll! (p. 41)

The Strange Case of Dr Jekyll and Mr Hyde is a treatise on the duality of man. Stevenson says in the voice of Dr Jekyll, '[T]hat Man is not truly one, but truly two. I say two, because the state of my own knowledge does not pass beyond that point. Others will follow, others will outstrip me on the same lines; and I hazard the guess that man will be ultimately known for a mere polity of multifarious, incongruous, and independent denizens' (p. 42).

Stevenson's proposition is that, perhaps, a separation of the two distinct elements of a person might secure a more harmonious entity rather than the conflicted and intractable curse of polar twins bound together yet struggling hopelessly. But even though there is no separate, embodied other, the suggestion is that the distinct elements might alter the body's form, in turn:

> Edward Hyde was so much smaller, slighter, and younger than Henry Jekyll. Even as good shone upon the countenance of the one, evil was written broadly and plainly on the face of the other. Evil besides . . . had left

on that body an imprint of deformity and decay. And yet when I looked upon that ugly idol in the glass, I was conscious of no repugnance, rather of a leap of welcome. (p. 44)

In this account, the dual aspects of the self have memory in common, but all other faculties were shared unequally. Stevenson anticipated the phenomenology of multiple personality disorder (dissociative identity disorder), emphasizing the unawareness of the personalities of the totality of each other's consciousness and memories. He writes in the voice of Dr Jekyll,

Jekyll (who was composite), now with the most sensitive apprehensions, now with a greedy gusto, projected and shared in the pleasures and adventures of Hyde; but Hyde was indifferent to Jekyll or but remembers him as the mountain bandit remembers the cavern in which he conceals himself from pursuit. Jekyll had more than a father's interest; Hyde had more than a son's indifference. (p. 48)

Karl Miller (1987) has said of Robert Louis Stevenson that he seemed 'to live out his fictions, for being the bourgeois drop-out who does not desert the fold, for camping out on Treasure Island. And casting himself away there at the head of a Scots Family Stevenson' (p. 212). The idea here is that Stevenson was aware of the differing aspects of himself, his duality, if you wish, and that this awareness lay at the heart of the novel, *The Strange Case of Dr Jekyll and Mr Hyde*. Stevenson also wrote a play, *Deacon Brodie, or The Double Life* which deals in the nature of the double as duality.

Deacon Brodie's (1741–1788) life embodied the duality of human nature. He was born in Edinburgh and was a prominent cabinetmaker by trade, crafting exquisite furniture for the city's elite. However, beneath this respectable veneer, he harboured a secret: his involvement in a life of crime and deception. Brodie's double life began to unfold in the late eighteenth century when he established a network of criminals and began carrying out daring burglaries throughout Edinburgh. Using his skills as a locksmith, Brodie developed intricate schemes to infiltrate the homes of the wealthy, pilfering their valuables under the cover of darkness. What made Brodie's crimes even more intriguing was the stark contrast between his respectable day-to-day persona as a respected tradesman and his nocturnal activities as a master thief.

Brodie's criminal endeavours grew in boldness and audacity as did his thirst for excitement and risk. His success seemed unparalleled, earning him the moniker 'The Prince of Thieves'. However, like many who live on the edge, Brodie's luck eventually ran out. In a tragic turn of events, Brodie's double life was unveiled when one of his accomplices turned informant, leading to his arrest and subsequent trial in 1788. Although initially hailed as a popular public figure due to his influential connections, Brodie's true nature became exposed to the citizens of Edinburgh. The revelation of his secret life as a criminal surprised many people.

Rick Wilson (2015) in his book *The Man Who Was Jekyll and Hyde* makes the point that one of the cabinets manufactured by Deacon Brodie stood at the foot of Robert Louis Stevenson's bed in New Town Edinburgh, a century after it was made, and he argues that Stevenson became obsessed by the Brodie story, particularly about the human capacity for a plurality of personalities to inhabit one body. Stevenson said of this, '... in the room in which I slept as a child in Edinburgh there was a cabinet – and a very pretty piece of work it was too – from the hands of the original Deacon Brodie' (Wilson, 2015, p. 19). In regard to the inspiration for *The Strange Case of Dr Jekyll and Mr Hyde*, Stevenson is reported to have said, 'I had long been trying to find a body, a vehicle, for that strong sense of man's double being which must at times come in upon and overwhelm the mind of every thinking creature' (quoted in Wilson (2015, p. 15)).

Echoing Karl Miller's notions that Stevenson's own awareness of his dark inner world was reflected in his portrayal of Dr Jekyll, Rick Wilson makes the case for this even more cogently, arguing that Stevenson had admitted in his letters for keeping a mixed company and that he often escaped to 'murky, sexy Old Town underworld', and engaged in his own secret life of narcotics, alcohol, and sexual decadence. And that while he was overtly respectable, he loved to frequent whores and thieves in the lower end of town (Wilson, 2015).

The description of Deacon Brodie, which appeared in the Edinburgh press, as given in the Sheriff Clerk's appeal for his arrest, on 12 March 1788, is reminiscent of Stevenson's description of Mr Hyde:

> WILLIAM BRODIE is about five feet four inches – is about forty eight years of age, but looks rather younger than he is – broad at the shoulders and

very small over the lojns – has dark brown full eyes, with large black eyebrows – under the right eye there is the scar of a cut, which is still a little sore at the point of the eye next the nose ... a sallow complexion – a particular motion with his mouth and lips when he speaks, which does full and slow, his mouth being commonly open at the time, and his tongue doubling up, as it were, shows itself towards the roof of his mouth – black hair, twisted, turned up, and tied behind, coming far down upon each cheek .... (Wilson, 2015, p. 13)

There remain questions to this day about whether Deacon Brodie and his accomplice's trial was fair and whether death by hanging was appropriate for crimes, no matter how heinous, which did not involve murder. Nonetheless, Deacon Brodie was hanged in public, before a crowd of over 40,000 people. Until the last moment, there were stories about the possibility of Brodie cheating death at the gallows, either by bribing the hangman or by collusion with the overseeing doctor to have a steel tube fashioned to protect his neck. It was also reported that, ironically, Brodie had been earlier involved in the redesign of the gallows at which he was hanged. In the end, he died by hanging on 1 October 1788. This ended the life of a burglar who was a member of the Town Council, Deacon of the Wrights (joiners, cabinetmakers, coffin makers), well off and well-born, a descendant of Morayshire lairds (Miller, 1987).

William Sharp and Fiona Macleod

The story of Deacon Brodie is important as much for its association with Stevenson's *The Strange Case of Dr Jekyll and Mr Hyde* as for the insight that it gives to the possibility of, indeed, the actuality of duality of personalities in human affairs. In this context, the emphasis is on the moral and behavioural polarities of the individual concerned, the respectable counterpoised against the dark and nefarious. The true story of William Sharp (1855–1905) provides a counterpoint to this narrative.

William Sharp was born on 12 September 1855, in Paisley, Scotland (Figure 4.2). He was a prolific writer, editor, and critic, and his works covered a wide range of genres including poetry, fiction, and biography. Sharp established himself as a respected figure in the literary world, but in

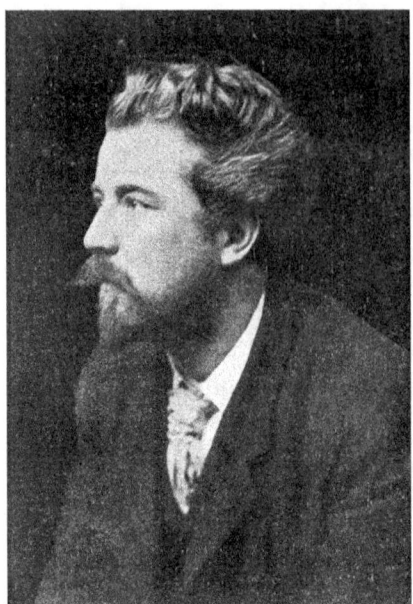

Figure 4.2 William Sharp 1855–1905 (Public domain)

1893, a new literary persona emerged – Fiona Macleod. Fiona Macleod was introduced as a female writer hailing from the Highlands of Scotland, and her writing greatly differed from that of William Sharp. However, Fiona Macleod was a pseudonym of William Sharp, a secret that was finally revealed upon his death. Although they were believed to be separate individuals during their time, it was eventually revealed that William Sharp and Fiona Macleod were the same person. Fiona Macleod's works were known for their lyrical beauty and their deep connection to nature, mythology, and the Celtic spirit. She explored themes of love, nature, spirituality, and the mystical elements of the Scottish landscape. Macleod's writings, on the other hand, had ethereal and haunting qualities, creating a unique blend of Celtic folklore and romanticism.

Sharp, under the guise of Fiona Macleod, published numerous volumes of poetry and prose. The works, such as *Pharais* (1894), which was dedicated to Edith Wingate Rinder, *Mountain Lovers* (1895), and *The Washer of the Ford* (1896), gained significant popularity for their evocative language and profound exploration of the human condition. Macleod's writing often explored the realms of the supernatural and mythical, blurring the lines between reality and fantasy.

Unlike Deacon Brodie, William Sharp and Fiona Macleod were the two sides of a multifaceted writer, one a male writer and the other a female writer. The first two novels by Macleod, *Pharais* and *The Mountain Lovers*, were commercially successful, and in the wake of their success, Sharp decided to invent a life for Fiona Macleod, and to present her personality through publications and letters. He promoted her writings, acted as her agent, asserted that she was a cousin, and implied to others that they were lovers. He moulded the persona of Fiona Macleod for a decade or so and sustained it with the assistance of his wife and cousin Elizabeth Sharp, his sister Mary Sharp who supplied Fiona Macleod's handwriting, Edith Wingate Rinder with whom he developed a strong bond, and Mona Caird, an independent woman married to a wealthy Scottish Laird (Halloran, 2022).

The female persona of Fiona Macleod was only the culmination of William Sharp's dual nature. Apparently, since childhood, he had assumed the guise of different people. This had been expressed in terms of mood, one William Sharp happy and outgoing and the other sad and bitter. Eventually, the duality came to be defined by the dominance of reason over emotion, and finally as being both a man and woman but with distinct personalities and outlooks. In a letter addressed to a friend Eric Robertson, accompanying a sonnet, Sharp wrote, 'There are two "William Sharps" – one of them unhappy and bitter enough at heart, God knows – though he seldom shows it. The other poor devil also sends you a greeting of his own kind [sonnet]' (Halloran, 2022, p. 26).

We know from Elizabeth Sharp, his wife and cousin, that William Sharp based Fiona Macleod on Edith Wingate Rinder and she wrote about this as follows:

> Because of her beauty, her strong sense of life and the joy of life; because of her keen intuitions and mental alertness, her personality stood for him as a symbol of the heroic women of Greek and Celtic days, a symbol, that as he expressed it, unlocked new doors in his mind and put him 'in touch with ancestral memories' of his race. So, for a time, he stilled the critical, intellectual mood of William Sharp to give play to the development of this

new found expression of subtler emotions, towards which he had been moving with all the ardour of his nature. (Halloran, 2022, p. 124)

William Sharp did suffer from depression, but there is no evidence of a direct link between the mood disturbance and the duality expressed in his writings. However, of course, the bouts of depression may very well have alighted him to the fact of the differing aspects of the self. He wrote to Elizabeth in 1891,

> I have been here all day and have enjoyed the bodily rest, the inner quietude, and latterly, a certain mental uplifting. But at first I was deep down in the blues. Anything like the appalling gloom between two and three thirty! I could scarcely read or do anything but watch it with a kind of fascinated horror. It is going down to the grave indeed to be submerged in that hideous pall. (Halloran, 2022)

Here we can glimpse something of his attitude towards his depressive bout – not so much resignation but a passive acceptance of the deadening experience of depression. On another occasion, writing to his friend Gilchrist who himself suffered from depression, in 1894, Sharp said,

> To be alive and young and in health is a boon so inestimable that you ought to fall on your knees among your moorland heather and thank the gods. Dejection is a demon to be ruled. We cannot always resist his tyranny, but we can always to become bondagers to his usurpation. Look upon him as an Afreet to be exorcised with a red-hot iron. He is a coward weakling, after all: take him by the tail and swing him across the moor or down the valley. Swing up into your best. Be brave, strong, self-reliant. Then you live. (Halloran, 2022, p. 133)

It is clear from the foregoing that the encounter with depression was one that was fraught with danger. There is a hint that life itself was at stake.

Summary

In this chapter, I have explored how the double motif as duality is expressed and represented in fiction. Stevenson's *Dr Jekyll and Mr Hyde* is the hallmark text as it aligns the duality in the individual with good and evil sides and furthers this by making corporeal the imagined difference. The good side being a respectable doctor, who is tall, and the evil side being Mr Hyde, who is small and unwholesome in appearance. I also draw attention to the real-life model for Stevenson's novel, in the person of Deacon Brodie who lived a public life as a civic leader and a secret and sinful life of crime. Finally, I examined the life of William Sharp and his pseudonym Fiona Macleod to demonstrate that duality need not be to do with the distinction between good and evil, but as we see in William Sharp's case, the distinction was between a male writer and his female alter ego. The male writer represented rationality, whereas his female alter ego stood for what was emotional.

CHAPTER 5

Implicit Double in Fiction

A name can be in any number of places: a person can only be in one place.

(Euripides c. 480–c. 406 BC)

I want now to turn to a different form of duality, one that does not involve an internal double, or what Rogers termed 'latent double', but rather operates on an implicit notion of the double that influences beliefs and behaviour (Rogers, 1970). This form of the double motif is exemplified in the clinical scenario in which an individual believes that a familiar person, such as a parent or spouse, has been replaced by impostors or robots. In spite of identical physical appearance, the individual is convinced that the familiar is no longer themselves. This conviction relies on the implicit belief that doubles are not only possible but also probable. There is also the related clinical situation in which an individual believes that a physically unfamiliar person is a familiar person who is masquerading. These clinical conditions are rarely represented in fiction, and when they are, the accounts are not typical of clinical cases. Yet, these accounts are worthy of our interest and scrutiny.

Ray Bradbury's 'The Martian'

Ray Bradbury (1920–2012) was an American novelist best known for his sci-fi novels and short stories. He is, perhaps, best known for *Fahrenheit 451* in which he depicts a dystopian world where books are banned and burned. In the *Martian Chronicles*, he writes a collection of interconnected stories about the arrival of humans on Mars. In one of the short stories 'The Martian', Bradbury writes about a Martian survivor who is capable of materializing, assuming any form that it desires. It materializes as Tom, the deceased son of LaFarge and his wife. Even though they both realize that the boy couldn't be Tom, their yearning was so great that they preferred this 'Tom' to not having him:

> 'Who are you, really? You can't be Tom, but you are someone. Who?' 'Don't.' Startled, the boy put his hands to his face. 'You can tell me,' said the old man. 'I'll understand. You're a Martian, aren't you? I've heard tales of the Martians; nothing definite. Stories about how rare Martians are and when they come among us they come as Earth Men. There's something about you – you're Tom and yet you're not.' 'Why can't you accept me and stop talking?' cried the boy. His hands completely shielded his face. 'Don't doubt, please don't doubt me!' He turned and ran from the table. (Bradbury, 2001, pp. 161–162)

This replica of the known Tom, but not quite, is reminiscent of the situation in Capgras syndrome where the patient believes that a familiar person has been replaced by an impostor. There is recognition but a failure of identification.

We learn later about a man, Mr Nomland, who had seen a man on Mars whom he had murdered while he still lived on Earth:

> 'All kinds of words tonight. You know that fellow named Nomland who lives down the canal in the tin hut?' LaFarge stiffened. 'Yes?' 'You know what sort of rascal he was?' 'Rumour had it he left Earth because he killed a man.' Saul leaned on his wet pole, gazing at LaFarge. 'Remember the name of the man he killed?' 'Gillings, wasn't it?' 'Right. Gillings. Well, about two hours ago Mr Nomland came running to town crying about how he had seen Gillings, alive, here on Mars, today, this afternoon! He tried to get the jail to lock him up safe. The jail wouldn't. So Nomland went home, and twenty minutes ago, as I get the story, blew his brains out with a gun. I just came from there.' (Bradbury, 2001, p. 163)

So, we have a variant of Proteus, maybe even a chameleon, on Mars, with the ability to become a simulacrum, investing the hopes and longings of memory with the corporeality that it lacked. In Capgras syndrome, there is the belief that a familiar other is replaced by an exact double and in Frégoli syndrome that a familiar other masquerades in an unfamiliar mask. This account by Ray Bradbury is different only insofar as Mr

LaFarge correctly recognizes that the Martian has materialized as a known other; in that respect, it is similar but not identical to Capgras syndrome, but we are yet to find what the original form of the Martian is. Bradbury continues:

> Who is this, he thought, in need of love as much as we? Who is he and what is he, that, out of loneliness, he comes into the alien camp and assumes the voice and face of memory and stands among us, accepted and happy at last? From what mountain, what cave, what small last race of people remaining on this world when the rockets came from Earth? The old man shook his head. There was no way to know. This, to all purposes, was Tom. (p. 164)

But the Martian himself said, 'I'm not anyone, I'm just myself; wherever I am, I am something, and now I'm something you can't help' (p. 168).

In this story, it is the desires and yearnings of human beings that determine the form that the Martian takes. And because of this character of the Martian, as it passes through a crowd, it metamorphizes into the dearest and most cherished memories of the individuals who make up the crowd: 'Across the open plaza leading to the landing, the one figure ran, It was not Tom; it was only a running shape with a face like silver shining in the light of the globes clustered about the plaza, And as it rushed nearer, nearer, it became more familiar, until when it reached the landing it was Tom!' (pp. 169–170).

But as a crowd surged around the Martian:

> Before their eyes he changed. He was Tom and James and a man named Switchman, another named Butterfield; he was the town mayor and the young girl Judith and the husband William and the wife Clarisse. He was melting wax shaping to their minds. They shouted, they pressed forward, pleading. He screamed, threw out his hands, his face dissolving to each demand, 'Tom!' cried LaFarge. 'Alice!' another. 'William!' They snatched his wrists, whirled him about, until with one last shriek of horror he fell. He lay on the stones, melted wax cooling, his face all faces, one eye blue, the other golden, hair that was brown, red, yellow, black, one eyebrow thick, one thin, one hand large, one small. (p. 171)

It is not merely that this story has aspects of Capgras syndrome, but it also has aspects of the delusion of intermetamorphosis, a condition in which, in real time, dynamic transformations take place with unfamiliar individuals transforming into familiar others. In the story of 'The Martian', the strain of continuous transformation is such that the Martian dies.

This type of double motif, which is expressed as duality, does not necessarily involve dual characteristics. There is no emphasis on the polarities of virtue or gender. There is no malfeasance or behavioural anomaly; simply being identical to an imagined other is sufficient. This capacity for protean transformation restores to life hopes and dreams or redeems loss or makes reparation for grief.

Patrick McGrath's Spider

Patrick McGrath is a British novelist known for his psychologically rich and Gothic-infused works that explore themes of madness, identity, and the darker aspects of human nature. He was born on 7 February 1950, in London. McGrath's own life experiences and family background have deeply influenced his writing. His father was Medical Superintendent of Broadmoor Hospital, a highly secure mental hospital. McGrath's childhood experiences, when he lived close to Broadmoor Hospital from the age of five, probably influenced his choice of literary subject and style.

McGrath's novels often feature unreliable narrators and probe the complexities of the human psyche. In *Spider*, McGrath delves into the mind of a disturbed protagonist named Spider, who grapples with memories of his traumatic childhood and struggles to distinguish between reality and delusion. The novel's exploration of mental illness and the subjective nature of memory earned critical acclaim and was later adapted into a film directed by David Cronenberg.

In another novel, *Asylum*, McGrath investigates the dark underbelly of a psychiatric hospital in post-war England. The story revolves around a forbidden romance between a psychiatrist's wife and a patient, exploring themes of desire, repression, and the boundaries between sanity and madness.

Patrick McGrath's (1990) novel *Spider* is a different take on the double. It examines the troubled mind of its protagonist, Dennis 'Spider' Cleg, as he grapples with his disturbing memories and unravelling grip on reality. The story takes place in London, where Spider, a middle-aged man recently released from a mental institution, is sent to live in a halfway house. As the narrative goes between Spider's present and past, McGrath explores themes of identity, memory, and madness.

Spider's crumbling mental state is evident from the start. As the unreliable narrator, he is haunted by fragmented memories, and his delusions gradually entangle his perception of the everyday world. He becomes fixated on his childhood home and the tragic events that occurred there, particularly the strained relationship between his parents. McGrath immerses readers in Spider's mind as he becomes increasingly mentally unwell and isolated. His perspective becomes fragmented and unreliable, making it difficult to separate truth from fiction.

The theme of duality runs throughout the novel. It is present at the very beginning of the novel:

> [T]he woman who runs the boarding house I'm living in (just temporarily) has the same last name as the woman responsible for the tragedy that befell my family twenty years ago. Beyond the name there is no resemblance. My Mrs. Wilkinson is an altogether different creature from Hilda Wilkinson, she's a sour, vindictive woman, big, it's true, as Hilda was big, but with none of Hilda's sauce and vitality, far more interested in questions of control . . . .
> (McGrath, 1990, p. 9)

It involves the narrator too: 'I haven't even told you my name yet! It's Dennis, but my mother always called me Spider' (p. 20). He is Dennis 'Spider' Cleg, a person with two aspects to him. And the Spider character could take on a different aspect too, sometimes as a protective mechanism when he was being physically abused by his father:

> Into this circle I stepped and began to unbutton the thick gray wool trousers that came down to my kneecaps and were held up by a pair of striped braces, which all boys wore in those days. The trousers would fall in an untidy heap about my boots, followed by my thick winter underpants, and then without a word I'd cross my arms on the beam and lean my head on them, and bend over the waist. I'd pretend then that there was a different Spider leaning against the beam, or even tied to the beam, or even *nailed* to the beam – with me taking the belt to *him*. Often I'd imagine my father nailed to the beam. (p. 53, emphasis in the original)

The doubling and complex set of identifications described demonstrates not only that Dennis is split off from Spider but also that, furthermore, there's a detachment from the Spider character to the degree that it is Dennis who is flogging Spider or even that it is the father who is being flogged by Dennis. There are hints here that the psychological process of dissociation that involves a separation of aspects of conscious awareness is at play here and that this may be severe enough to correspond to depersonalization. This process is often reported by individuals who have experienced significant psychological trauma such as childhood physical and/or sexual abuse.

There are rich and enthralling depictions of psychotic experiences in *Spider*. Sometimes, it is impossible to distinguish between mere play of imagination and delusional beliefs that determine how the world is imagined, perceived, and interpreted. To complicate matters, there are also visual and other hallucinatory experiences. Since the story is being told by Spider, and much of the account relies on memory, which is itself subject to distortion and falsehood, the reader's understanding is confounded and under constant assault.

Spider believes that he witnessed his mother's murder by his father and that the woman whom he identifies as Hilda Wilkinson was present at the time of the murder. He wakes up and goes down to the kitchen,

> I opened the door. My father was sitting at the table with a woman I had never seen before. 'What is it?' he said. 'What's the matter with you?' He rose to his feet and led me out of the kitchen into the passage, closing the door behind him. 'Back upstairs', he said, guiding me down the passage. 'back to bed, Dennis'. . . . 'Where's my mum?' I cried. 'I don't want to go back to bed, I had a dream!' 'That's enough', he said, pushing me down the passage. 'I want my mum!' 'Don't make me angry, Dennis! Your mum's in the kitchen'. 'No, she's not!' (p. 79)

Spider examines this other woman, Hilda Wilkinson, and says of her smell, 'this too was a woman's smell, but it was Hilda's smell, a warm, fleshy smell coloured by strong perfume and emanations of her fur, which, impregnated with fog, hung from the wardrobe door. There was also the smell of her feet, and the whole effect was of some large female animal, not terribly clean, possibly dangerous' (p. 82).

And there are differences, too, to be found in Hilda Wilkinson's physique and in the way that she moves, to differentiate her from Spider's mother:

> I watched her pick her way carefully down our narrow stairs, descending in a cautious sideways movement in a tight-belted dark blue dress with small spots: *my mother's Sunday dress*. I watched her go down, her bottom bulging and a plump hand on the banister, and as I listened to the clack of her heels I couldn't help remembering the soft slushy shuffling sound my mother's slippers made when she moved around the house. She had painted her mouth with my mother's lipstick and fixed her hair with my mother's comb; the scent, however, was all Hilda. (p. 84, emphasis in the original)

In Capgras syndrome, there is a conviction that despite physical identity, the misidentified individual is an impostor. Sometimes, there are minor, trivial reasons for suspecting duplication: the voice is different in tenor, the gait or standing stance is minutely different, or the use of words is said to be unusual. In Spider's case, though, he was confident that there were gross physical differences between Hilda Wilkinson and his mother:

> I think what distressed me most after Hilda moved into number twenty-seven was seeing my mother's clothes being worn by a prostitute. It was not only the idea of trespass and violation, there was the daily spectacle of what happened to the clothes when Hilda put them on. My mother was a slender woman, she had slim, delicate figure, boyish almost, whereas Hilda was all curves, she was *fleshy*. So my mother's clothes were tight on her, and became as a result provocative; what had been demure on my mother was tarty on Hilda, but then that was the nature of the woman, everything she touched in some way became tarty. (p. 114, emphasis in the original)

The doubling also involves his psychiatrist, Dr Jebb, whom he identified with his father:

> I was staring straight into eyes the same cold shade of blue as my father's! I shrank back in my chair (a hard wooden one). He had the same hair as my father, black, lank, and oily, combed straight back off a narrow forehead and flopping about his temples: he frequently pushed a hand

through it when he frowned. The same narrow nose, the same pencil-thin moustache neatly hedging the top lip, the same wiry build and tone of pent explosive energy. (p. 185)

And there is also the doubling of place, the identification of Canada with Ganderhill – one an imaginary and unreal place, named after a country, and the other an asylum that is described with exactitude. There is, in addition, the trigger of old memories by the kitchen at Hilda Wilkinson's boarding house, a type of reduplication of place that evolved into a transformation of Hilda Wilkinson, the landlady of the boarding house, into the Hilda Wilkinson character who is misidentified as his mother's impostor:

> But what riveted my attention to this brightly lit scene, framed as it was in the kitchen door at the end of that short dark passage, was the way she handled the roller, the way she rose up on her toes and *leaned* on the thing so that all the strength and weight of those beefy shoulders was transmitted down her powerful arms, through her wrists, and into the thick fingers of her hamlike hands, the nails of which, I saw with a very thrill of recognition and horror, and despite the powdering of flour upon them, were *filthy*. For a moment past and present slid seamlessly together, assumed identity, and there was *one woman* only leaning on that rolling pin, and that woman was Hilda Wilkinson; at that moment the woman in the kitchen was transfigured, her hair was blonde with black roots, her bosom strained against the fabric of an apron not her own, and her sturdy legs were planted on the kitchen floor like a pair of tree trunks ... *Her chin*! How could I have missed it? She had Hilda's chin, big and puggy, *prognathous*, the very same! 'Ah, Mr. Cleg', she said – and I was back in 1957 with my landlady once more. (pp. 128–129, emphasis in the original)

It is often said that jealousy is a disturbance of the eyes, of looking, of the gaze. Anyone afflicted with jealousy looks and studies every movement, every facial expression, and the nuance of every social interaction, imbuing them with meaning and assumed intentions and motivations. In *Spider*, there is a precision of description of the visual world, reminiscent of pathological jealousy. And this is understandable, given that visual recognition of persons is fraught with potential error: the most subtle of features signal the difference between originals and copies. Spider is attentive to the most mundane of physiognomic characteristics as he is to the features of rooms and landscapes. It is as if he would lose his bearing, his foothold even, if minute discrepancies were not urgently and immediately grasped.

Even the Spider character has a plenitude of doubles:

> [O]ver the years Spider has learned that it is often necessary to allow Dennis to face the world, or 'Mr. Cleg' for that matter; not only this, but intermediate compartments have become necessary – with Dr. McNaughten, for instance, who knows my history. The front of my head does not satisfy the doctor so he is permitted contact with what used to be the back of my head but is now the chamber occupied by a Dennis Cleg with 'my history' – but Spider's never there! Spider's elsewhere, though the doctor suspects nothing. (p. 135)

In another scene, Spider says, 'So, while I entered the room as Spider of London, I stepped out of it a lunatic, unrecognizable to myself' (p. 167). The name Spider is itself a metaphor both of his ability to ensnare others into his web as well as of vulnerability, his weakness, and fear of being ensnared.

The novel culminates in a shocking and poignant revelation that Spider killed his mother, and that he was put away in an asylum for the crime of matricide. The novel is constructed in such a way that the reader discovers the dark secret of the novel at the same time that Spider also comes to recognize his role in his mother's death. This is as powerful a novel we will ever get, which subjects the reader to the manipulations and distortions of a psychotic imagination, of the compelling inner logic of psychosis, of delusions, more precisely. The novel forces readers to question their own perceptions and assumptions. It centres on the Capgras syndrome, the misidentification of a familiar person as unfamiliar, as other. This belief drives the narrative thrust of the novel and makes comprehensible the matricide. The extent of Spider's psychosis is profound and plausible. I have argued that often the verisimilitude of the description of abnormal psychopathology is rooted in personal experience. There is no evidence that Patrick McGrath has experienced abnormal phenomena. However, his father was Medical Superintendent of Broadmoor Hospital, a high-security hospital, in Britain, for the care of mentally ill offenders, and he grew up near Broadmoor. Hence, the fidelity of his descriptions to the actuality of psychosis and to asylum life is probably due to this experience.

The novels and short story that I have dealt with in this chapter open a different kind of exploration of the double motif. In the previous chapter, in Stevenson's hands, we have a single character with dual and conflicting personalities. Each personality informs the structure of bodily habitus, and the propensities and attitudes of each personality are distinct and opposite. In Ray Bradbury's story, the double motif is expressed in the embodiment of the hopes, memories, and aspirations of people in the vicinity of the Martian. Here, the double is usually of a person already deceased and missed by relatives. In McGrath's novel, the double motif is expressed in multiple ways but principally in the misidentification of a familiar person, Spider's mother, for another person, Hilda Wilkinson. This misidentification has tragic consequences, but the internal logic is comprehensible even if depraved.

Both *The Strange Case of Dr Jekyll and Mr Hyde* and *Spider*, have been made into films. Indeed, *The Strange Case of Dr Jekyll and Mr Hyde* has been made into several films: from 1920 onwards by John S. Robertson, in 1931 by Rouben Mamoulian, in 1942 by Victor Fleming, and in 1971 by Roy Ward Baker. *Spider* was made into a film by David Cronenberg in 2003.

Nabokov's Despair

Vladimir Nabokov was born on 22 April 1899, in Saint Petersburg, Russia (Figure 5.1). He was a novelist, poet, translator, and lepidopterist whose literary achievements spanned continents and languages. He is best known for his novels, which are characterized by their intricate prose, playful experimentation with language, and exploration of themes such as memory, identity, and the nature of reality much like many of the other novelists referred to in this book.

Nabokov's early life was marked by privilege and upheaval. He was born into a wealthy and aristocratic family and grew up in a cultured and multilingual environment. However, the Russian Revolution of 1917 and the subsequent turmoil forced the Nabokov family into exile. They fled to Crimea and later settled in various European cities before eventually emigrating to the United States in 1940, where Nabokov would spend

DOPPELGÄNGER: ANALYSING 'DOUBLES'

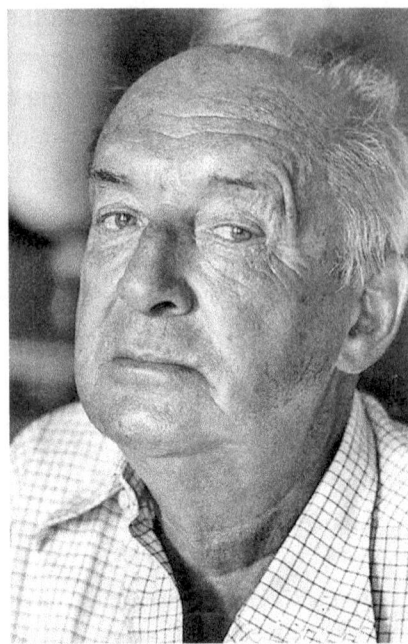

Figure 5.1 Vladimir Nabokov 1899–1977 (Public domain)

much of his life. Nabokov's literary career began in the 1920s with the publication of his first poems and short stories in Russian emigre journals. His early works, written in Russian, showcased his talent for lyrical prose and vivid imagery. However, it was his transition to writing in English that would catapult him to international acclaim.

Nabokov's breakthrough came with the publication of his novel *Lolita* in 1955. A controversial and audacious work, *Lolita* tells the story of Humbert Humbert, a middle-aged literature professor who becomes infatuated with his twelve-year-old stepdaughter, Lolita. The novel's exploration of taboo subjects such as paedophilia and its use of an unreliable narrator challenged conventional notions of morality and narrative technique. Despite its controversial subject matter, *Lolita* received critical acclaim for its linguistic virtuosity, psychological depth, and dark humour.

Vladimir Nabokov's (1966) *Despair* is a different type of account of the double. It is a complex novel narrated by Hermann, whose account is obviously unreliable. Nabokov said of Hermann,

> Hermann and Humbert [the central character of *Lolita*] are alike only in the sense that two dragons painted by the same artist at different periods of his life resemble each other. Both are neurotic scoundrels, yet there is a green lane in Paradise where Humbert is permitted to wander at dusk once a year; but Hell shall never parole Hermann. (p. 11)

The novel was first published in 1934 in the original Russian and translated into English by Nabokov himself in 1936 and published in 1937. The definitive English edition, edited by Nabokov, was published in 1965. *Despair* is regarded as one of his earlier and lesser-known works, yet it exhibits the themes and literary devices that would come to define his later masterpieces. In *Despair*, Nabokov weaves a tale of deceit, insanity, and the duality of human nature.

The novel follows the life of Hermann Karlovich, a successful and meticulous Russian businessman with a troubled mind. Hermann becomes convinced that he can commit the perfect crime: he will murder a man who bears a striking resemblance to himself and then assume the victim's identity, thereby escaping his mundane existence. This concept of doubles plays a significant role throughout the narrative, exploring the complexities and consequences of identity manipulation and self-deception.

In exploring Hermann's psychology and his inner life, Nabokov shows how hard it can be to distinguish between disturbed thinking, reality itself, and the morbid motivation that drives behaviour. Hermann is convinced that his planned murder is clever and perfect and that he has outsmarted everyone around him, including the reader. However, his schemes prove to be flawed and predictably so, and his desperate attempts to maintain the facade of normalcy eventually crumble under the scrutiny of those around him.

The narrative structure employed in *Despair* is as intricate as its theme. The story is presented through the unreliable perspective of Hermann himself, blurring the boundaries between reality and his distorted perception. Nabokov's writing navigates between Hermann's inner thoughts, his explicit storytelling, and his attempt to deceive the reader, creating an added layer of suspense and irony. Throughout the novel, Nabokov's *Despair* is not merely a fictional account utilizing the double motif but a suspense thriller, a crime novel, and a display of the wonders of language. The prose is elegant and precise, borrowing from and often adapting the Russian classic literature of Pushkin and Dostoyevsky. As with many of his works, Nabokov showcases his multicultural and multilingual background, incorporating references to German and Russian literature as his facility with French, and wordplay that adds richness to the narrative. Furthermore, *Despair* is an examination of the nature of storytelling, and the relationship between fiction and deception, raising questions about the nature of truth and the ways in which individuals shape their own narratives.

In *Dr Jekyll and Mr Hyde* (see Chapter 4), we saw how the distinct aspects of a person's psyche can shape, even deforming the body to suit the dark and criminal self. In this story, there is no discrete and separate embodied other. In *Spider*, in the context of severe mental illness, probably schizophrenia, an implicit notion of the double shapes the inner logic – the disturbed, irrational logic that fuels the aberrant conviction that Spider's mother has been replaced by an impostor. In *Despair*, there is no double who is a part of the original, but another person who happens to look like our protagonist. This is the most overt manifestation of the double motif. Hermann finds his physical doppelgänger, Felix, who bears a remarkable resemblance to himself. Hermann becomes fixated on the idea of murdering Felix and stealing his identity, effectively becoming his own double. This resemblance is the basis of the plan to commit murder. But there are other uses that Nabokov puts the double motif to.

Alongside the physical resemblance, Hermann also senses a mysterious connection with Felix on a psychological level. He believes that they share the same thoughts, emotions, and desires, further fuelling his desire to replace Felix and take on his identity. Nabokov blurs the line between the reader and the character, implicating the reader in the unfolding narrative so that, in a sense, the reader becomes a double for Hermann. Hermann addresses the reader directly, attempting to manipulate their perception of events and presenting himself as a sympathetic protagonist. This implicates the reader as an accomplice in Hermann's web of deceit, effectively becoming his unseen double.

The novel itself mirrors the concept of a double through its narrative structure. Hermann serves as the unreliable narrator, his version of events often differing from the reality presented. This duality adds intrigue and challenges the reader's perception of truth, effectively creating a narrative double within the story. And finally, the concept of identity plays a central role in *Despair*. Hermann's desire to assume Felix's identity represents a larger theme of individuals grappling with their own identity. The novel explores the idea of self-deception and the willingness to adopt another's persona to escape the restrictions of one's own existence.

So, to summarize, *Despair*, unlike the other (McGrath's *Spider*), showcases two independent individuals who look alike. In this, it is closer to Saramago's *Double* than it is to the other novels that I have treated so far. In both, the affinity between the two people is determined by physical identity, and, therefore, the novels allow an exploration of what it is that determines psychological identity and how this differs from physical identity. There is also always the question of precedence – of who it is, who the original is, and who the copy is. Hermann says:

> Our resemblance struck me as a freak bordering on the miraculous. What interested him was mainly my wishing to see any resemblance at all. He appeared to my eyes as my double, that is, as a creature bodily identical with me. It was this absolute sameness which gave me so piercing a thrill. He on his part saw me as a doubtful imitator. (p. 21)

Hermann also makes the point that it is the face in repose, in sleep, and possibly in death that is most identical. The idea here is that the living face, life as lived, mars the apparent identity in much the same way that 'a breeze dims the bliss of Narcissus' (p. 22).

In *Dr Jekyll and Mr Hyde* (see Chapter 4), a story that is a literary exemplar of dissociative identity disorder (multiple personality disorder) introduces the concept of the process of dissociation as a possible psychological mechanism that underlies pathological displays of identity disturbance. Nabokov takes this idea forward and uses it to explain how Hermann feels during the act of sexual intercourse with his wife:

> Not only had I always been eminently satisfied with my meek bedmate and her cherubic charms, but I had noticed lately, with gratitude to nature and a thrill of surprise, that the violence and sweetness of my nightly joys were

being raised to an exquisite vertex owing to a certain aberration which, I understand, is not as uncommon as I thought at first among high-strung men in their middle thirties. I am referring to a well-known kind of 'dissociation'. With me it started in a fragmentary fashion a few months before my trip to Prague. For example, I would be in bed with Lydia, winding up the brief series of preparatory caresses she was supposed to be entitled to, when all at once I would become aware that imp Split had taken over. My face was buried in the fold of her neck, her legs had started to clamp me, the ashtray toppled off the bed table, the universe followed – but at the same time, incomprehensibly and delightful, I was standing naked in the middle of the room, one hand resting on the back of the chair where she had left her stockings and panties. The sensation of being in two places at once gave me an extraordinary kick; but this was nothing compared to later developments. (p. 32)

Later, Hermann acquired the skill to sit apart at a distance from the sexual action, watching, as it were, himself engaged in sex. Indeed, he describes having a sensation of greater ecstasy the longer the interval, the distance between the two selves such that he longed to discover some means to remove himself at least a hundred yards from the lighted stage where he performed. Here we have the splitting of the self into two, a distancing of the self from the scene of action and not necessarily a momentary process but sometimes so involved that the link between the agentic self and the observing self became tenuous and precarious. On one occasion, the observing self inhabited a phantasmal world where Hermann thought that he was in bed with Lydia when in fact he was seated in a chair.

This is a form of the double motif that we have not previously encountered. The splitting that occurs in *Dr Jekyll and Mr Hyde* (see Chapter 4) was determined by a secret potion invented by Dr Jekyll, whereas in *Despair*, Nabokov relied on a naturally existing psychological mechanism that was described by Pierre Janet (1859–1947), a French psychiatrist in the nineteenth century. Dissociation is often associated with traumatic experiences in childhood, a process that allows the core self to be protected from the cruelty and harmful consequences of unfathomable physical cruelty and horrific sexual abuse.

Hermann experiences, transiently, an autoscopic vision: '... there appeared a form, that of a man ... the moment he reached me, or, better, say, he seemed to enter into me, and pass through, as if I were a shadow' (p. 51). So, *Despair* is replete with different forms of the double: the physical double, the dissociated double, the mirrored double, and so on. Hermann develops a preoccupation with mirrors – an aversion to mirrors, more properly speaking. This preoccupation has a season when he admired his own reflection, while surveying himself in mirrors, then a period ensued when he avoided mirrors because the reflected image had a negative, if not perplexing, connotation. There is also the use of his fingers to trace the outline of his face yet without recognition. It is therefore not just that a visual mirror image is not satisfying, but a tactile image of his familiar face is unrecognizable.

Déja vu experiences are an example of anomalous phenomena. They are, typically, phenomena whereby an individual has a strong sense that unfamiliar or novel events or places have been previously experienced; they are the evocation of familiarity in the context of the unfamiliar. Fundamentally, these experiences speak to the nature and mechanisms for experiencing a sense of duplication, or, to put it in another way, these experiences force us to consider how a breakdown of the neurological mechanism that notates an event or place as unique occurs and is then manifest as a phenomenon in conscious awareness. Hermann says:

> Well do I remember that little town – and feel oddly perplexed: should I go on giving instances of such aspects of it, which in a horribly unpleasant way echoed things I had somewhere seen long ago? It even seems to me now that it was, that town, constructed of certain refuse particles of my past, for I discovered in it things most remarkably and most uncannily familiar to me. (p. 66)

In *Jamais vu*, the reverse occurs – an individual has a deep sense of the unfamiliar, of strangeness or alienation in a context that ought to be familiar. These experiences are associated with the delusional misidentification syndromes, the central plank of Patrick McGrath's novel *Spider*.

It could be argued that *Despair* is an exploration of the notion of the double in all of its intricacies. It includes the idea of a theatrical understudy, a double, even if he or she is surplus to requirements. Hermann refers to these understudies as 'star ghosts' and brings into play the idea of substitution, the same underlying rationale that patients invoke as an explanation for their belief, in Capgras syndrome, that close relatives have been replaced by impostors; the patient would say, 'they've been substituted!'.

Despair is self-consciously a novel about the double. Hermann, our unreliable narrator, says:

> What amazed me was the absence of title on the first leaf: for assuredly I *had* at one time invented a title, something beginning with 'Memoirs of a –' of a what? I could not remember; and anyway, 'Memoirs' seemed dreadfully dull and commonplace. What should I call my book then? 'The Double'? But Russian literature possessed one already. 'Crime and Pun'? Not bad – a little crude, though. 'The Mirror'? Too jejune, too à la mode ... what about 'The Likeness'? 'The Unrecognised Likeness'? 'Justification of a Likeness'? .... (pp. 167–168)

For all the effort to commit the perfect murder based on the likeness between two people, one of the concluding thoughts is, 'It is not enough, however, to kill a man and clothe him adequately. A single additional detail is wanted and that is: resemblance between the two; but in this whole world there are not and cannot be, two men alike, however you disguise them ...' (p. 170). Here, the conclusion seems to be a disavowal of the foundations of the crime as well as of the novel itself.

Summary

In this chapter, I introduced the idea of the implicit double. This approach to the notion of the double works, precisely because there is an idea, an implicit notion that doubles exist or can exist. So, Bradbury, McGrath, and Nabokov exploit this belief in various ways. In Bradbury, the double provides rescues from grief and loneliness, in McGrath, it provides the ground for matricide, and in Nabokov, it is the basis for a plot to carry out a perfect murder.

In the following chapter, I examine how the double motif is dealt with in films, investigating the varied approaches to the double motif in cinema and the novel. There are cinematic resources, dependent as they are on the visual, the auditory, and the creative use of mood, atmosphere, and tempo, which are unavailable to the novelist. These resources that cinema brings to the task allow for a shift in the nature of narrative structure, of how plot and time can be differently manipulated, and of how reality, fantasy, and mental derangement can be represented.

CHAPTER 6

The Double in Film

So, gentlemen, a Being, some new Being which, like ourselves, will undoubtedly multiply and increase, is now on earth. What? Why are you smiling? Because the Being is till invisible? But, gentlemen, what a primitive organ is the eye! It can barely spot our basic needs for survival. It misses the infinitesimal as well as the infinite.

(Guy de Maupassant 1850–1893)

Film has the technical resources and the visual possibilities to facilitate the portrayal of stories that rely on the double motif. Perhaps, Alfred Hitchcock, the British film-maker, was the best and most notable exponent of the double motif in film. Alfred Hitchcock is widely regarded as the Master of Suspense, and was born on 13 August 1899, in Leytonstone, London, England (Figure 6.1). Hitchcock's career began in silent film during the 1920s, where he worked as a title designer, art director, and eventually a director. His early films like *The Lodger* (1927) showcased his unique ability to create tension and atmosphere, setting the tone for his future works. It wasn't until the 1930s that he gained international recognition with movies like *The 39 Steps* (1935) and *The Lady Vanishes* (1938). In the 1940s, Hitchcock moved to Hollywood, where he had his golden age as a film-maker. He crafted a series of suspenseful and psychological thrillers, including *Shadow of a Doubt* (1943), *Notorious* (1946), and *Strangers on a Train* (1951). However, it was his 1960 film *Psycho* that solidified his status as a cinematic genius. The shower scene in this movie, along with its shocking narrative twist, became iconic and greatly influenced the horror genre.

There are several examples of the double motif in Hitchcock's films including *Shadow of a Doubt* (1943), *Strangers on a Train* (1951), *The Wrong Man* (1957), *Vertigo* (1958), and *Psycho* (1960). In these films, Hitchcock

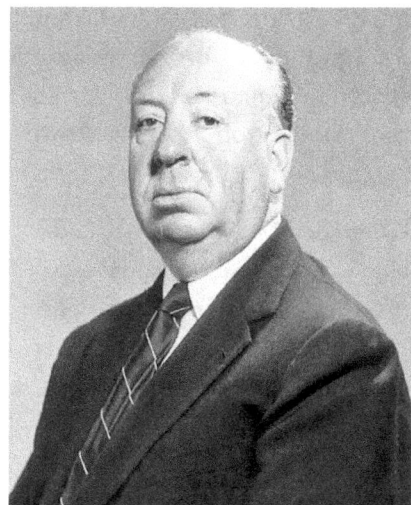

Figure 6.1 Alfred Hitchcock 1899–1980 (Public domain)

explores themes of duality, deception, and the psychological aspects of identity.

Shadow of a Doubt (1943) tells the story of a young girl named Charlie (played by Teresa Wright) who is eagerly anticipating the arrival of her charming Uncle Charlie (Joseph Cotten) from out of town. However, her excitement quickly turns to suspicion when she begins to suspect that her uncle may be a notorious serial killer on the run. As the story progresses, the tension between Charlie and her uncle builds as she tries to get to the bottom of his true intentions. Her suspicions are further heightened when two detectives arrive in town to investigate the series of murders, and she finds herself caught between her loyalty to her uncle and her growing fear that he may be a dangerous killer.

Shadow of a Doubt is widely regarded as one of Hitchcock's finest works, and for good reason. From the opening scenes, Hitchcock builds an atmosphere of paranoia and suspicion that keeps the audience on edge throughout the entire film. The performances by Wright and Cotten are both outstanding, with Wright's Charlie portraying a complex mix of innocence and determination as she tries to uncover the truth about her uncle.

Hitchcock employs the double motif in this film. Uncle Charlie represents a dark mirror image of his niece's own inner struggles. So, this is a film that counterpoises the innocence and vulnerability of Wright's Charlie against the dark, dangerous, and ruthless Cotten's uncle Charlie. As Donald Spoto has pointed out,

> The structural element at work in Shadow of a Doubt … is the almost infinite accumulation of doubles: the two Charlies; two detectives in the East pursuing Uncle Charlie, then the two in West; two criminals sought; two women with eyeglasses; two dinner sequences; two amateur sleuths engaged in two conversations about killing; two young children; two older siblings; two railway sequences; two sequences outside a church; two doctors; two double brandies served at the 'Till Two' bar by a waitress who has worked there for two weeks; two attempts to kill the girl before the final scene; two scenes in a garage, one a declaration of love and one an attempt at murder – and so on, almost past counting. (Spoto, 1984, p. 263)

Here is an example of the use of the double as a filmic device, a tool to deepen the viewers' interest in the notion of doubling, and I suppose to raise attention and expectation to certain aspects of the story. This is a latent double motif. Uncle Charlie and Charlie are counterposed. There is little subtlety in Uncle Charlie, his character is ruthless and deceptive, and there is an absence of duality in him except that his debonair exterior is cover for the ruthless undertow. There is a hint in Wright's Charlie of her recognition that there are aspects of herself that may be like that of Uncle Charlie. She says, 'We are both alike' and again 'we are like twins'. Despite these statements, she is more light than darkness.

In *Strangers on a Train* (1951), Hitchcock continues his fascination with the double motif. The film follows the tale of two strangers who meet by chance on a train and become embroiled in a sinister pact. The story revolves around two central characters: Guy Haines (Farley Grainger), a talented professional tennis player who dreams of a successful career, and Bruno Antony (Robert Walker), a mysterious and disturbed man with a fascination for murder. Guy finds himself trapped in an unhappy marriage to the manipulative and unfaithful Miriam, while Bruno harbours deep-seated resentment towards his overbearing father.

On a train ride, Bruno confronts Guy with an unsettling proposition. Based on a theory he has developed, Bruno proposes that they swap murders – Bruno will kill Guy's wife, freeing him from his troubled marriage, and Guy will murder Bruno's tyrannical father, thereby granting Bruno the freedom he craves. Shocked and horrified, Guy dismisses the idea as absurd and quickly distances himself from Bruno.

However, Bruno does not let go so easily. In a calculated move to bind Guy to their agreement, he stalks Miriam and eventually carries out the murder himself, making it appear as if Guy had orchestrated the deed. Consumed by guilt and fear, Guy now finds himself trapped in a web of Bruno's creation.

Guy becomes increasingly desperate to withdraw himself from Bruno's scheme, fearing that he would come under suspicion. The audience is held captive by Hitchcock's signature mastery of suspense. The tension builds to a crescendo during a climactic scene at a carnival, where Guy fights to reclaim his freedom, clear his name, and bring justice to Miriam's killer.

Strangers on a Train addresses complex themes of guilt, deception, and the lengths to which people will go to achieve their desires. Guilt is central to many of Hitchcock's films. The mere association with the murder of Miriam induces a sense of guilt in Guy, and this in turn makes his behaviour suspicious, a fact that is not lost on the policemen who have him under surveillance. The film explores the capacity for murder in human beings and our seeming fascination with crime and murder. Bruno says, 'Everybody is a potential murderer'.

There is Hitchcock's style of employing the double motif in film: there are, at the very beginning of the film, two pairs of feet and two sets of train rails that cross twice. Guy and Bruno meet when their crossed feet accidentally touch under a table, and Bruno orders a pair of double drinks. There are two respectable and influential fathers, two women with eyeglasses, and two women at a party who enjoy thinking up ways of committing the perfect murder. There are two sets of detectives in two cities, two little boys on the two trips to the fairground, two old men on the carousel, two boyfriends accompanying Miriam to the fairground, and two Hitchcocks in the film. Hitchcock, the director, makes his cameo appearance, carrying a double bass fiddle onto the train.

The film is adapted by Raymond Chandler and Czenzi Ormonde from a Patricia Highsmith novel. In the novel, there is no reference to the double motif, an aspect of the film added by Hitchcock himself. Donald Spoto (1984) makes the point that Hitchcock was familiar with E. T. A. Hoffmann's *Devil's Elixir*, Heinrich Heine's *Ratcliff*, Edgar Allan Poe's 'William Wilson', and Dostoyevsky's *The Double*. Yet, in the film, there is no doubling of any person. There is no duality in either Guy or Bruno. They are both distinct, and as Spoto says,

> [Bruno] inhabits a world of darkness, marked by the shadows that crisscross his face, the Gothic gloominess of his Arlington mansion, and the boat Pluto that he takes to commit murder and that relates him to the god and household of the dead; he is the counterpart of Grainger [Guy], who inhabits the world of light, represented by bright open-air tennis games, light-coloured attire, and formal Washington dinner parties. (p. 328)

Nonetheless, Barbara Morton, in the part played by Patricia Hitchcock, is a doppelgänger of Miriam as both wear glasses and are petite. Indeed, Bruno is thrown when he first sees Barbara Morton, and on the second occasion while demonstrating what it is like to strangle someone, he sees her again and he loses control of himself to the degree that he almost kills the woman on whom he is demonstrating what it is like to strangle someone. Barbara Morton correctly guesses that he wishes to kill her but is ignorant of the underlying reason for this.

The Wrong Man (1957) is based on a true story, and the film opens with Alfred Hitchcock speaking to the camera and telling the audience that this film is based on real events. The protagonist, Manny Balestrero (Henry Fonda), is a devoted family man who plays bass in a jazz combo at a nightclub – The Stork Club, in New York City.

One day, he needs to borrow money to pay for his wife's dental work and decides to go to the insurance office where his wife had a life insurance policy. While there, the clerks recognize him as the man who had robbed the same office twice before. Manny Balestrero is arrested and charged with the crimes. Manny's wife, Rose (Vera Miles), is convinced of his innocence. She is emotionally and financially drained by the trial process, and the stress of the situation begins to take a toll on her mental health to the degree that she becomes profoundly depressed and requires hospital treatment. Despite the evidence in his favour, the case continues to move forward, and Manny is forced to endure the humiliating and dehumanizing experience of being imprisoned and put on trial for a crime he didn't commit. The climax of the film takes place in the police station. The true robber is arrested and correctly identified. Both he and Balestrero meet in the corridor of the police station, in a scene where Balestrero meets his doppelgänger. There is an uncanny similarity in their physical identity, with their similar height, weight, bone structure, and gait. But, nonetheless, they are distinguishable.

In preparing for the making of the film, Hitchcock took Henry Fonda and Vera Miles to meet the Balestrero family in Florida, where they had relocated after Rose was discharged from the hospital. Hitchcock also met with William B. Groat, the judge who had tried the case and who confirmed the details of the mistrial. A juror, Lloyd Espenschied, rose up during the trial and said to the judge, 'Judge, do we have to listen to all this?' – a question which implied that the juror had already made up his mind of the defendant's guilt. This was a breach in the protocol that a juror will refrain from any conclusion until he had heard all the evidence. This led Frank O'Connor, who had defended Balestrero, to file for a mistrial. It was during this interval that the real culprit was captured while attempting another robbery.

The plot of *The Wrong Man* worked on the hypothesis that Balestrero's arrest and ordeals were determined by mistaken identity and, by implication, that he had a doppelgänger. This was a marked departure from Greco-Roman comedies where the doppelgänger allowed for comic interactions and situations. What Hitchcock had happened upon was the possibility that a doppelgänger can also allow for tragic consequences and for pathos, for the evocation of pity and sadness. Tragedy works best when the reversal in fortune is undeserved, and it was totally undeserved in Balestrero's case. But, in addition to this, the film was a dramatization of a true story, and the double motif was further accentuated by the fact that the opening segment had Hitchcock telling the audience this fact and distinguishing *The Wrong Man* from his previous films, the distinction between fact and fiction. So, we have a doubling effect: the Balestrero family were being enacted on screen by actors, as were all the other protagonists including the real culprit. Lurking in the periphery of the viewer's mind is the degree to which the actors resembled the real people they were enacting.

Behind the scenes, there was a personal drama unfolding for Hitchcock. Spoto describes it as follows:

> Vera Miles was being detained by Hitchcock for eight to nine hours daily, trained and put through the poignant scenes of her breakdown over and over again until she was nearly sick with exhaustion. The situation began to resemble the control Carl Dreyer had exerted over Renee (Maria) Falconetti in *The Passion of Joan of Arc* three decades earlier, although in Hitchcock's case the control was never physically abusive, and in Vera Miles' case the breakdown never crossed from acting to reality, as in the case of the unfortunate Falconetti. Nevertheless, there was an atmosphere of Svengali and Trilby. (Spoto, 1984, p. 379)

The relationship between Hitchcock and Vera Miles had started well enough with Hitchcock sending her two dozen American Beauty roses each day with strangely ardent greetings, which she is said to have destroyed immediately. The Warner Brothers archives record daily story conferences with Vera Miles, but the content of these conferences is unknown except that Vera Miles was in a state of angry resentment. Vera Miles married Gordon Scott during the shooting of the *The Wrong Man*. From then to the end of the shooting, Hitchcock's relationship with Vera Miles cooled. This pattern of Hitchcock's desire to control, indeed, to domineer his leading ladies was manifest in the plot of *Vertigo*.

In *Vertigo* (1959), Hitchcock gives a doppelgänger a central role. *Vertigo* is a classic thriller starring James Stewart and Kim Novak. The film follows Scottie Ferguson (James Stewart), a retired San Francisco police detective who is asked by an old friend to investigate his wife, Madeleine (Kim Novak), who he believes is possessed by the spirit of a dead ancestor and is in danger of harming herself. As Scottie investigates, he falls in love with Madeleine and becomes obsessed with her, but she ultimately falls to her death from a church tower. Distraught and haunted by her memory, Scottie becomes melancholic and is admitted to the hospital.

Months later, Scottie encounters a woman named Judy (Kim Novak) who bears a striking resemblance to Madeleine. He soon realizes that

Judy was Madeleine's impersonator and was part of an elaborate plan to fake her death. As Scottie and Judy grow closer, he begins to manipulate her appearance and behaviour to resemble Madeleine more closely, as part of his ongoing obsession. However, the truth eventually comes to light. The film concludes with a dramatic sequence in which Scottie pursues Judy up the same church tower where Madeleine fell, leading to a tragic end.

Vertigo is widely regarded as an iconic film that explores themes of identity, obsession, and deception. The Madeleine character sits in front of a painting of Carlotta Valdes at the local museum. In the portrait, Carlotta holds a bunch of flowers, as does Madeleine, and they are wearing a frock of a similar colour, and their hairdos are similar. So, here Madeleine is sitting in front of her doppelgänger, her supposed ancestor, who is said to have killed herself. Judy and Madeleine are the same person and are both played by Kim Novak. After Madeleine's death, Scottie meets Judy and he becomes obsessive about her appearance and compels her against her wishes to dress like and to transform herself into Madeleine. This transformation includes changing her hair colour to blond.

I have argued that Dostoyevsky and Guy De Maupassant probably based their descriptions of autoscopy on personal experience. There is no description of autoscopy in *Vertigo*, but Spoto argues that Hitchcock's biography is relevant and important for *Vertigo*. There is a sense in which the obsessive transformation of Judy into Madeleine mirrored Hitchcock's obsession with the dress and demeanour of his leading ladies both in the characters that they were playing as well as in their personal lives. This meticulous attention to the detail of their appearance was true for Ingrid Bergman, Grace Kelly, Kim Novak, and Vera Miles. It culminated in his disastrous relationship with Tippi Hedren who resisted his attempts to rule her life and appearance outside of the film set.

This domineering attitude that Scottie had towards Judy's clothes, hairstyle, make-up, and manner was identical to Hitchcock's domineering attitude towards Kim Novak outside of the time and space of the film set. This, in essence, is an example of doubling: what was being portrayed in the film reflects Hitchcock's fantasy about the possibility of romance with his leading female characters. In this regard, James Stewart was

Hitchcock's alter ego, and Kim Novak, both in the film and in life, was a desirable but unattainable love object for Hitchcock. Hitchcock says of his comparison between women and suspense, '[Suspense] is like a woman. The more left to the imagination, the more the excitement ... The conventional big-bosomed blonde is not mysterious. And what could be more obvious than the old black velvet and pearls type? The perfect "woman of mystery" is one who is blonde, subtle and Nordic ...' Quoted in Spoto (1984, p. 398).

And in relation to the transformation of Judy to Madeleine, Hitchcock remarks,

> I was very much intrigued by the basic situation of Vertigo, ... – of changing the woman's hair colour – because it contained so much analogy to sex. This man changed and dressed up his woman, which seems like the reverse of stripping her naked. But it amounts to the same thing. I really made the film in order to get through to this subtle quality of a man's dreamlike nature. Quoted in Spoto (1984, p. 399)

Donald Spoto concludes that the man that Hitchcock was referring to was himself and that Hitchcock could not respond to a woman until she was refashioned to correspond to his dream.

It is in *Psycho* (1960) that Hitchcock finally deals with a story in which the character exemplifies the double motif rather than that filmic devices taking advantage of the double motif are at play. The story begins with Marion Crane, a young secretary from Phoenix, Arizona, who is discontented with her life and is in a forbidden relationship with a man, Sam. In a moment of desperation and impulsivity, she steals $40,000 from her employer and heads out of town to start a new life with Sam. But along the way, she stops at the Bates Motel, run by the strange and introverted Norman Bates, who appears to live with his overbearing mother in a house on the hill behind the motel. After a conversation with Norman about his mother, Marion begins to second-guess her decision to leave town and decides to return the money and confess her crime. However, before she can, she is brutally murdered in the shower by who we believe to be Norman's mother. Marion Crane's disappearance sets off a search by her sister, Lila, and Sam, who are aided by a private investigator. As the investigation continues, more and more secrets about Norman and his mother are uncovered, leading to a climax at the Bates Motel. We eventually learn that Norman is suffering from a severe case of split personality (dissociative identity disorder), where his 'mother' is actually a personality created by Norman to cope with his abusive upbringing. We also learn that Norman has been acting as both himself and his mother, carrying out a series of murders from the Bates Motel. In the end, Norman is captured, and it is revealed that he would not serve prison time but will be sent to a psychiatric institution. The final scene shows a shot of Norman, smiling as he thinks about 'his mother' conversing with him in his head.

Hitchcock's *Psycho* features prominent and various double motifs throughout. The double motifs are expressed through various elements of the narrative, including the two central characters, Marion Crane and Norman Bates, who are both shown to be struggling with their inner conflicts and divided selves. Other examples of doubles in *Psycho* include the fact that Marion steals money and Norman subsequently steals her corpse, as well as the visual symbolism of mirrors and reflections that are used to create a sense of duality and inner turmoil of the characters. Overall, the use of doubles in *Psycho* adds depth to the story and heightens the psychological tension, making it one of Hitchcock's most memorable and influential films.

Guilt is central to the story:

> Everyone in *Psycho* has a disguise or something to hide – the hidden treasure; the furtive plans of lunchtime lovers at the opening; wedding day tranquilizers secretly taken by Janet Leigh's co-worker [Marion Crane] Pat Hitchcock in her last role for her father; the bottle of whiskey hidden by the possessive father (Frank Albertson); the bottle of whiskey hidden in an employer's desk; the secrets of illicit affairs, stolen cash, concealed identities, and undiscovered murders. (Spoto, 1984)

Mirrors, too, are important. In this film, mirrors accentuate feeling. For example, Marion Crane looks at herself in the mirror, and we see her reflection at moments of uncertainty and of palpable feelings of guilt. On other occasions, the mirrors examine the nature of personal identity by revealing the duality in human nature. We see through the mirrors Marion's dual identity; the trustworthy Marion and the guilty and untrustworthy Marion who has stolen money. In addition to this use of mirrors, Donald Spoto draws attention to the different geometries that Hitchcock uses to create symbols of fractured personality in *Psycho* – the title designs of Saul Bass of bisecting horizontals and verticals, and the contrast of the horizontal motel and looming vertical house on the hill. Spoto says, 'The cutting imagery establishes a visual design in which conflict in the viewer extends to the conflict within the characters' (Spoto, 1984, p. 422).

In the final segment of *Psycho*, the psychiatrist provides an explanation for Norman Bates's problems. According to the psychiatrist, Norman suffers from split personality. He explains that Norman had created an alternate personality to cope with his intense feelings of guilt of killing his mother and her partner, and to escape the responsibility for his violent actions. The psychiatrist delves into the details of Norman's dissociation, stating that he created an entirely separate identity for his mother, Norma Bates. This identity eventually took over Norman's consciousness, causing him to believe that he and his mother were two distinct individuals. Norman's dissociation was so severe that he would often lose memory of his actions while assuming the persona of his mother. Furthermore, the psychiatrist argues that Norman's mother's personality took control whenever he felt threatened. It was this alter ego that committed the murders, not Norman himself. The psychiatrist concludes that Norman's belief of his mother's continued presence was a defence mechanism to shield him from the guilt and consequences of his actions.

In summary, the psychiatrist explains that Norman Bates's problems stem from a psychiatric condition, whereby he developed an alternate personality as a defence mechanism against guilt and responsibility. The psychiatrist (Simon Oakland) explains to Sam, Lila, and the authorities that Norman and his mother are two halves of a split personality. 'Norman Bates no longer exists', he says. 'He only half existed to begin with, and now, the other half has taken over, probably for all time'. Norman's incestuous desire for his mother led him to poison her when she took a lover, but guilt over the matricide obsessed him and compelled him to dig up her corpse and preserve it using his skills at taxidermy. But even this wasn't enough, so he had to create the illusion that his mother was alive by wearing her clothes and speaking in her voice. 'He was never all Norman', the psychiatrist explains, 'but he was often only mother, and now the dominant personality has won'. A final scene shows Norman alone, speaking in his mother's voice, totally dominated by his maternal persona (Meehan, 2017, p. 54). This view is summarized in the statement, 'When the mind houses two personalities, there's always a conflict, a battle'.

It could be argued, as the psychiatrist does in the film, that Norman Bates suffers from multiple personality disorder (dissociative identity disorder) and that *Psycho* is a filmic update of Robert Louis Stevenson's *Dr Jekyll and Mr Hyde*.

What are the resources unique to cinematography that are deployed in depicting the double motif? Fiction relies on the imagination of the reader to bring to life the story, whereas cinema depicts vividly and visually not only the plot but also the psychological mood and tempo of events. What can only be hinted at, obscurely, in literature can call our attention readily and compellingly, in film, such that we come to feel and to respond to manifest and as well to hidden meanings. The double motif, in Hitchcock's hands, evolved in such a way that it is not merely the use of a doppelgänger that we experience but the accentuation of our feelings by the doubling of objects with the use of mirrors and duplication by cinematography. And Hitchcock's use of the double motif is inextricably linked with his favourite theme, murder. It is always for him an exploration of the fertile grounds on which murderous instincts germinate, a probing of the psychological setting of murder or at the very least of sin and guilt.

Hitchcock was not the first film-maker to use the double motif, nor was he the last. *The Student of Prague* (1913) was the first feature-length horror film that featured a doppelgänger, and Fritz Lang in *Metropolis* (1927), which was set in 2026, introduced a robot doppelgänger Maria. Three of the novels discussed in Chapter 3, Dostoyevsky's *The Double* (2013) (directed by Richard Ayoade), Saramago's *The Double*, adapted as a psychological thriller *Enemy* (2013) (directed by Denis Villeneuve), and Stephen King's *The Dark Half* (1993) (directed by George Romero), have all been made into films.

It is in the development of sci-fi films that the use of the double motif has blossomed most – from Fritz Lang's *Metropolis* (1927) through to such films as *The Perfect Woman* (1945), *It Came from Outerspace* (1953), *Invasion* of the *Body Snatchers* (1956), *Forbidden Planet* (1956), *I Married a Monster from Outerspace* (1958), and *The Far Side of the Sun* (1969). It is Tarkovsky's *Solaris* (1972) that takes an imaginative leap forward in the use and treatment of the doppelgänger. The film is based on the novel *Solaris* by Stanislaw Lem (1987).

In Stanislaw Lem's *Solaris*, the story focuses on the mysterious and enigmatic planet Solaris. The book examines themes of human consciousness, perception, and the limitations of scientific understanding. The narrative begins on a space station orbiting Solaris, where a team of scientists has been studying the planet for years. The scientists are perplexed by the planet's unique abilities, as it seems to possess a massive living ocean that has the power to materialize physical manifestations of the scientists' hidden thoughts and memories. The protagonist, psychologist Kris Kelvin, travels to Solaris to assess the mental well-being of the scientists on the space station. Upon arrival, Kelvin discovers that the scientists have fallen into deep emotional distress due to the mysterious phenomena occurring on the planet. They have encountered 'guests', physical replicas of people from their past, appearing as if conjured out of their memories. These guests evoke deep emotional responses in the scientists and challenge their understanding of reality.

Kelvin himself encounters a guest, a version of his late wife, Rheya, who had died by suicide years earlier. The reappearance of Rheya forces Kelvin to confront the unresolved guilt and love he felt for her. As Kelvin grapples with these complex emotions, he becomes increasingly immersed in the planet's unsettling and incomprehensible nature. Throughout the story, the narrative raises deep existential questions and explores the complexity of the human mind. Lem examines the limitations of scientific knowledge, suggesting that the boundaries of understanding the universe cannot be defined through conventional methods alone. He emphasizes the transient nature of human perception and the difficulty in comprehending the true nature of reality.

As Kelvin and his fellow scientists continue their studies, they realize that their attempts to communicate with and comprehend Solaris are futile. The planet's living ocean appears to be aware of their efforts and responds by creating increasingly perplexing and inexplicable phenomena. It becomes evident that Solaris is beyond human comprehension, an entity with a consciousness that defies conventional understanding.

Kelvin's interactions with the replica of Rheya become increasingly tumultuous. He struggles to accept her as anything but a mere reflection of his own memories, leading to intense moments of psychological and emotional turmoil. The story examines the challenging nature of confronting one's personal demons. In the end, Kelvin reaches a realization that humanity's limited understanding of the universe prevents them from fully comprehending and communicating with entities like Solaris. He acknowledges the futility of continuing to study the planet and gives up hope of ever unlocking its mysteries. The novel culminates in an open-ended conclusion, leaving readers with a sense of wonder and contemplation.

Stanislaw Lem's *Solaris* challenges conventional ideas of perception, reality, and scientific understanding. Through Kelvin's experiences on the space station, the novel paints a portrait of human complexity and the limitations of knowledge. It invites readers to contemplate the nature of consciousness, the boundaries of human comprehension, and the fundamental nature of reality itself.

The novel *Solaris* and Andrei Tarkovsky's film adaptation of the same name share the same core story and explore similar themes, but they differ in significant ways. In the novel, the main character is Kris Kelvin, a psychologist who confronts his own emotional turmoil and guilt through his interactions with the doppelgänger of his late wife on the space station. Tarkovsky's film, however, shifts the focus from the personal journey of Kelvin while exploring broader philosophical and existential questions. As a film-maker, Tarkovsky used the medium of cinema to create a distinct visual and atmospheric experience. The film incorporates long takes, slow pacing, and deliberate cinematography to evoke a sense of contemplation and immersion. Lem's novel, on the other hand, relies on descriptive prose to convey the otherworldly nature of Solaris and the characters' experiences.

Lem's novel is a traditional narrative with a linear progression, following the events on the space station and Kelvin's emotional journey. Tarkovsky's film, however, deviates from a straightforward storytelling approach. It includes extended dream sequences and abstract imagery, blending past and present, reality and memory, to capture the psychological and metaphysical aspects of the story. Furthermore, while Lem's novel explores the scientific inquiry and attempts to understand Solaris, the planet, Tarkovsky's film downplays the scientific elements. It departs from the more explicit scientific inquiries and explanations found in the book, focusing more on the philosophical and metaphysical aspects of human existence and consciousness. Finally, Tarkovsky's film places a greater emphasis on exploring the characters' inner lives and their relationships with one another. The film dives deeper into the emotional complexities and psychological struggles of the scientists, emphasizing the impact of their encounters with the mysterious guests from Solaris.

It's important to note that while both the novel and the film share the same central themes and ideas, Tarkovsky's adaptation takes artistic liberties to create a unique cinematic experience. Each medium offers its own distinct interpretation of Solaris, resulting in different narrative approaches and visual styles. Both the novel and the film stand on their own merits and contribute to the rich exploration of the profound questions raised by Lem's concept of Solaris.

Paul Meehan's judgement of the film is that

> [T]he film is slow-paced, talky, overlong, dull and pretentious. The screenplay by Tarkovsky and Fridrikh Gorenshtein takes much of the focus away from the novel's theme of the futility of communicating with an enigmatic alien intelligence and instead becomes merely a dramatic study of a failed marital relationship. There are long stretches of dialogue that digress into abstract philosophical discussions and pointless character backstory. On the plus side, the curvilinear space station sets are at once pleasing to the eye and claustrophobic and the visuals are smoothly photographed by cameraman Vadim Yusov. (Meehan, 2017b, p. 162)

Nonetheless, Tarkovsky's film won the Grand Prix at Cannes in 1972 and was nominated for the Palme d'Or.

It is *The Matrix* (1999), directed by the Wachowskis, that brings the doppelgänger motif into the digital age. The story takes place in a dystopian future where machines have enslaved humanity by creating a simulated reality called 'The Matrix' to distract humans from the real world. The film follows the journey of Thomas Anderson, a computer programmer by day and a notorious hacker by night, who goes by the alias 'Neo'.

Neo (Keanu Reeves) is someone who senses that there is something wrong with the world and is constantly searching for answers. His suspicions about the nature of reality are confirmed when he encounters a group of rebels led by the enigmatic Morpheus (Laurence Fishburne). Morpheus and his crew believe that Neo is 'The One', a prophesied figure destined to liberate humanity from the machines. Morpheus offers Neo a choice between a red pill and a blue pill, symbolizing the decision to either embrace the truth or continue living in the comfortable illusion of The Matrix. Neo chooses the red pill and is awakened to the harsh reality: humans are being used as mere energy sources by the machines, while their minds are trapped inside The Matrix.

As Neo begins his journey to understand his new reality, he meets Trinity (Carrie-Anne Moss), a skilled martial artist and member of Morpheus's crew. Trinity believes in Neo's potential and forms an emotional connection with him. Together, they set out to rescue Morpheus, who has been captured by Agent Smith (Hugo Weaving), a sentient program within The Matrix determined to maintain the status quo. Under Morpheus's captivity, Agent Smith attempts to break his mind and discover the codes that provide access to the mainframe of the human resistance. Meanwhile, Neo and Trinity plan a daring rescue mission. They enter The Matrix, where they encounter mind-bending challenges, engaging in battles against powerful computer-generated adversaries.

The film showcases groundbreaking visual effects, as Neo learns to bend the rules of The Matrix to his advantage, defying the laws of physics. As he exploits his abilities as 'The One', he becomes unstoppable. Alongside Trinity and Morpheus, Neo confronts Agent Smith in a showdown, displaying extraordinary skills and a willingness to sacrifice himself for the greater good. In a final battle, Neo transcends his limitations and achieves a state of true enlightenment, becoming a superhuman figure capable of reshaping reality itself. With his newfound powers, Neo defeats Agent Smith and frees humanity from The Matrix. As the film concludes, Neo makes a choice to save humanity but is left with a lingering feeling that the struggle against the machines is far from over.

The Matrix captivated audiences with its innovative storytelling, mind-bending concepts, and vivid action sequences. The film explores themes of reality and identity, prompting viewers to question their own existence and the nature of the world around them. Its success spawned two sequels, *The Matrix Reloaded* and *The Matrix Revolutions*, which further developed the complex narrative of The Matrix universe.

The Matrix has made a lasting impact on popular culture, influencing numerous films, video games, and works of art. Its philosophical undertones and thought-provoking themes continue to resonate with audiences, making it a key milestone in the sci-fi genre. Part of its success was determined by cinematic technology devised by John Gaeta. The film employed a technique called 'bullet time' that combined slow motion cinematography with 360-degree camera movement to create the illusion of the characters dodging bullets in flight. This was achieved using an array of super slow-motion cameras arranged in a circle around the subject and fired simultaneously. Another innovation was the use of 'wire work', already invented by Asian film-makers. Actors are suspended by an elaborate system of wires that create the illusion of levitation or flying. These techniques helped the film win Oscars in the special effects category. Despite its influence and success, there are critics who point to the glorification of violence and gunplay in *The Matrix*.

There are several double motifs in *The Matrix*. The Matrix is itself a simulacrum of a late-twentieth-century city designed to keep humans pacified and distracted within a system of neural activation. In other words, The Matrix resembles reduplicative paramnesia, a variant of delusional misidentification syndrome (see Chapter 1) in which a person holds the false belief that a place has been duplicated. Of course, The Matrix is different insofar as the inhabitants are unaware that they live in a simulation. Next, human beings are held within a womb-like pod, with cables attached to various parts of their bodies. Their day-to-day experiences and behaviours are enacted through doubles existing within The Matrix. The rebels, led by Morpheus, can penetrate the virtual reality of The Matrix by using a plug at the back of their heads. This allows them to operate within The Matrix, as doubles of themselves, or to use the language of the film, as 'residual self-image'. While in the virtual reality, their bodies remain in a coma in the real world. However, if the person dies within The Matrix, they also die in the real world. Hence, Morpheus remarks, 'The body cannot live without the mind, your mind makes it real'.

Paul Meehan describes the doppelgänger aspect as follows:

> In the filmic reality of *The Matrix* the double is presented as a digital construct, a simulacrum of the body connected with sleep and the world of dreams. While the body sleeps the doppelgänger is propelled into a virtual realm where it possesses magical powers. This idea ultimately derives from ancient shamanic and psychic practices having to do with bilocation and out of body experiences. There is also a connection with the phenomenon of 'lucid dreaming', in which the dreamer becomes aware he is dreaming and can influence events within the dream, and the name 'Morpheus' is a reference to the Greek god of sleep. In an early scene in the film, Anderson quips, 'ever get that feeling where you're not sure if you're awake or still dreaming?' The Keanu Reeves character has a dual identity as 'Anderson' inside the Matrix and 'Neo' in the real world, and although he completely transitions into the Neo identity, he is always referred to as 'Mr. Anderson' by Agent Smith. Note that Morpheus, Trinity and the other characters that enter the Matrix do not have this dual identity. (Meehan, 2017b, p. 186)

In the sequel, *The Matrix Reloaded* (2003) doppelgängers proliferate. Agent Smith is able to duplicate himself into infinite numbers of doppelgangers and The Twins (Neil & Adrian Rayment) are played by identical twins who wear identical white outfits, have bleached white dreadlocks and can materialise and de-materialise at will.

Avatar (2009), directed by James Cameron, invented the use of motion capture techniques combined with stereoscopic filming and digital animation. It was in the vanguard of 3D filming. The film is set in the year 2154, when humanity has already ventured beyond Earth to the distant planet of Pandora in search of a valuable mineral called unobtanium. This mineral promises enormous wealth, but it can only be found within Pandora's lush and vibrant ecosystem, inhabited by a race of tall, blue-skinned beings called the Na'vi. The story follows

Jake Sully (Sam Worthington), a paraplegic former Marine who takes part in the Avatar Program, a project that allows humans to remotely control genetically engineered bodies that resemble the Na'vi. Jake's twin brother, a scientist, was part of the project, but tragically died, leaving Jake with the opportunity to take his place.

As Jake arrives on Pandora, he is initially overwhelmed by its beauty and the wonder of his new avatar body. In the company of Dr Grace Augustine (Sigourney Weaver), a researcher studying the Na'vi, and Colonel Miles Quaritch (Stephen Lang), the head of security, Jake begins to explore the planet and the Na'vi way of life. While tasked with gathering information on the Na'vi and their connection to the Hometree, the heart of their culture, Jake's undercover mission soon takes an unexpected turn.

During a scouting mission, Jake encounters Neytiri (Zoe Saldana), a young Na'vi woman, and their meeting marks a turning point in his allegiance. Neytiri recognizes Jake as a warrior destined to bring balance and harmony to Pandora. She becomes his guide, teaching him about their culture, spirituality, and deep connection to the planet's ecosystem.

As Jake comes to understand the Na'vi way of life, he becomes torn between his loyalty to the human expedition and his affection for Neytiri and her people. He witnesses the destructive actions of the human corporation, led by Parker Selfridge (Giovanni Ribisi), which is ruthless in its exploitation of Pandora, jeopardizing not only the Na'vi but the very balance of the planet's ecosystem. Driven by his new-found connection to Pandora and the Na'vi, Jake decides to join their fight against the humans. He learns to embrace the Na'vi way, going through a rite of passage and becoming integrated into their society. Together with Neytiri and other Na'vi warriors, Jake leads a resistance movement against the human forces, determined to protect Pandora and its people.

In a decisive battle, the Na'vi stand against the formidable human military and their advanced technology. The Na'vi are joined by other creatures of Pandora, including giant flying creatures called banshees, and the iconic direhorse; they fight for their land, their culture, and their way of life. Ultimately, the unobtanium-rich Hometree is destroyed, but Jake's transformation and the resilience of his new-found family signal hope for a future beyond human greed and destruction.

The film ends with the defeat of the humans and the restoration of balance to the planet. As Jake permanently transfers his consciousness into his avatar body; he becomes a part of Pandora, forever dedicated to protecting its beauty and preserving the harmony between the Na'vi and the planet's ecosystem.

Avatar is not just a visually stunning and technically important film; it explores themes of environmentalism, colonialism, and the importance of cultural respect. Its message resonates with audiences, reminding us of the interconnectedness of all living beings and the need to protect the natural world we inhabit.

There is much in *Avatar* that builds on the notion of the double in *The Matrix*. As Paul Meehan puts it,

> The avatar concept has certain similarities with the digital doppelgänger depicted in the *Matrix* movies. In both films the protagonist uses a machine that links the protagonist to an alternate version of themselves while their bodies lie inert in a dreaming state. Their doubles can then perform superhuman feats while inhabiting a fantastic alternate reality. In *Avatar*, Jake Sully comes to prefer his existence in a bio-engineered artificial body to his life as a cripple in the human world as actor Sam Worthington becomes increasingly upstaged by his motion-captured, computer-generated onscreen alter ego. The film connects the double with shamanic dream states as recorded in the folklore of pre-industrial cultures and with the present-day phenomenon of 'lucid dreaming'. The motif of Jake having to replace his identical twin brother as an avatar driver is another reference to the doppelgänger concept. (Meehan, 2017b, p. 199)

Summary

In this chapter, I have focused on the films of Alfred Hitchcock, Tarkovsky, the Wachowskis, and James Cameron. The double motif has been explored, extended, and invigorated by cinema. Right from the beginning of cinema, in the silent era, through to the present day, with the extraordinary advances in technology that facilitate further development and enhancement of the dramatization of the double motif, stories employing the motif have continued to thrill, entertain, and enthral audiences.

There is a way in which cinema is itself a realm of doubles. Images of actors are captured and duplicated and then shown in theatres for our pleasure and edification. This is, in many respects, the magic of photography and of cinematography. Images can stand in for us, detached and distinct from the original. Our participation, as audiences, in the cinema requires us to enter the world of the film, to believe in the simulacrum that is created, so compellingly vital and true-like that for a moment we forget our everyday reality. Perhaps, this is a measure of why the doppelgänger motif is so powerful and so ubiquitous.

CHAPTER 7

The Double in Clinical Psychopathology

I have a little shadow that goes in and out with me,
And what can be the use of him is more than I can see.
He is very, very like me from the heels up to the head;
And I see him jump before me, when I jump into bed.

(Robert Louis Stevenson 1850–1894)

So far, I have reviewed the place of the double motif in antiquity, in fiction, and in cinema. I have shown how ubiquitous the double motif is across cultures and historical time. The variants include the physical duplication of persons, a metaphorical use of the double motif, and the implicit notion of the double as a means of dealing with the complexity of the human psyche. I have argued that the closer the description of the double is to the examples seen in psychiatric clinics, the more likely it is that the writer has personal experience of the pathological phenomena that are the models for the literary and cinematic uses of the double motif.

I want now to turn to the clinical phenomena that are likely to be the basis of the varied and intriguing literary and cinematic examples of the double motif. These include autoscopy and related phenomena, dissociative identity disorder (multiple personality disorder), and delusional misidentification syndromes. These clinical conditions are profound disturbances that affect the sense of psychological integrity, the unity of the self and body, and notions of personal identity and the identity of others. I will take each in turn.

Autoscopy and Related Phenomena

McConnell (1965) described a case of autoscopy in 1965 in which a pregnant woman said,

> I see myself just as I am, in clothes I'm wearing. It comes out of the blue when I least expect it and it would stagger you. It's the front view as if in a mirror. It's just a second or two. I turn away quickly whenever I see it and when I look back it's gone. It's just me and I don't do a thing.

The double was said to be dressed exactly as the patient. The double was solid and not transparent and was a mirror image. The patient found the double to be pleasing, and over time the double diminished to merely a vision of the upper body and then of the face alone.

This is an example of autoscopy, which involves the pure visual experience of seeing one's own body or its upper parts as if reflected in a mirror. It is significant that what the patient sees is often, but not always, a mirror image of the self. The vision is in natural colours and is usually motionless or may imitate the gestures, movements, or facial expressions of the patient.

Brugger et al. (1997), the leading authorities on the subject, describe six main types of autoscopy. The main types include autoscopic hallucination, heautoscopy proper, feeling of presence, out-of-the-body experience, negative heautoscopy, and inner autoscopy.

Heautoscopy proper, like autoscopy, involves seeing the double, but, in addition, there may be other kinds of experiences including a feeling of detachment from the double, strange and anomalous sensations of the body such as feelings of lightness and occasionally the experience of vertigo. The double may appear transparent, grey, or ghost-like. The double may imitate the patient's actions but may also act autonomously, not necessarily mirroring the patient's actions or movements. The characteristics of the double may differ from the patients such that it might be smaller or bigger, younger or older, and the gender may not be congruent with that of the patient. And surprisingly the patient may feel that he can see the world through the eyes of the double.

Jean Lhermitte described it as follows:

> Sometimes the hallucinatory image appears very thin, as if it were a projection on the screen; at other times, on the contrary, it would seem to be made of jelly-like or glass-like substance, so that the patient can see everywhere around him through this ghostly illusion, which would be impossible if the image were real. This is not a constant rule, and often

the phantom seems to be made of an opaque substance, not transparent to the eye.

The term 'feeling of presence' describes a feeling of the physical presence of oneself or of another person who is not seen but appears to be just out of sight. The patient may, in addition, experience altered or anomalous sensations in their body. Lukianowicz described a case of a man in 1967 who said,

> Sometimes I *feel* with the special feeling of a blind man approaching a wall, or with the extra sense of a man who feels his way in a pitch-dark room, my 'other self' moving about a foot in front of me or beside me. I have never seen him with my eyes, but I feel him around me and sometimes when I sit down I feel that I am resting on my own, or so to say, on my 'double's' knees. After a while our two bodies merged into one again ....
> (Lukianowicz, 1967, emphasis in the original)

Out-of-the-body experience involves seeing one's body from an outside perspective. The core of this experience is the separation of the body from the experiencing self. Typically, the inert body is observed from a detached and an elevated spatial position. The body is usually motionless during the observation. The surrounding environment is also seen from an elevated perspective. There is an associated strong emotional accompaniment and significance to the experience, and the emotions are more often positive except in cases where the experience is a precursor to a seizure. Lunn described a case in 1970 of a soldier who, in 1944, had sustained a shell injury to the left side of his head. Shell splinters were removed from the right parietal region (Lunn, 1970). The patient described his experience as follows:

> Suddenly, it was as if he saw himself in the bed in front of him. He felt as if he were at the other end of the room, as if he were floating in space below the ceiling in the corner facing the bed, from where he could observe his own body in the bed. The episode lasted for several minutes, ample time for the details to be impressed on his mind; he saw his own completely immobile body in the bed; the eyes closed. He noted the large [medical] dressing (which he had often seen in a mirror), the colour of the hair, the pale complexion. The experience seemed real; for the duration of the

episode, he felt convinced that he was watching his own dead body. He failed to detect the respiration and was fully convinced that he had died. The vision terrified him, he was struck dumb with horror; consequently, he could not communicate with his roommates. Throughout the episode, he distinctly heard their voices coming from 'below', his own self being suspended in space. He felt positive that he had been fully conscious throughout. The vision had gone as abruptly as it had come. Afterwards, he had palpitations, and it was sometime before he realized that he was still alive.

Negative heautoscopy refers to the failure to perceive one's own body in a mirror or when looked at directly. It is often accompanied by depersonalization and the loss of awareness of one's own body, sometimes termed aschematia. Negative heautoscopy can be unilateral, affecting only the perception of one half of the body. The most quoted example is from Guy de Maupassant's *The Horla*, which is, of course, a fictional account but given credence because Guy de Maupassant is reported to have experienced autoscopy:

> So there I was, pretending to this presence which I knew was spying on me that I was reading. All of a sudden I felt it reading over my shoulder, brushing against my ear. Leaping to my feet, I turned round so quickly that I nearly fell over. Believe it or not, though the room was bright as day, there was no sign of me in the mirror. It was empty, clear and full of light. But my reflection was not in it, despite the fact that I was standing directly in front of it. I looked at the large glass, clear now from top to bottom. I looked at it in terror..... (Maupassant, 2004)

However, there is a less graphic but nonetheless instructive case described by Villiers Lunn (1970) in 1970. This was a young man who had sustained a traumatic head injury to the right parietal region with subsequent epilepsy, right-sided weakness, and loss of sensation. He described the following:

> Suddenly, he felt as if he were standing with folded arms, leaning over the end of the bed. He could distinctly feel the pressure across his chest. He saw his own silent, motionless body in the bed: 'I looked very pale and emaciated and I could not help thinking that I must be very ill if I look so

bad'. He was extremely upset by the experience but, by a big effort of will, had managed to pull himself out of this 'split personality' state ... Two days before, he experienced the following: he was driving in his car to visit some friends. Suddenly, it was as if his left arm had gone leaving in its place a 'gap', almost as if his arm had been cut off at the shoulder. The sensation had been very realistic and, horrified, he had felt with his right hand to discover what had happened. He had felt much relieved when he found that everything was all right. The sensation had lasted for two hours and was equally intense throughout.

Finally, inner/internal heautoscopy refers to the experience of visual hallucination of one's own internal organs outside the body. Rao described a case in 1992 of an elderly man with a depressive episode who reported

> that he could 'see' his brain as a lotus coloured pinkish mass of flesh with grooves and bulges. He further stated that it was covered by a layer of smoke. He expressed surprise over this phenomenon agreeing that it is impossible for a person to see his internal organ. He claimed he could recognize his brain, based on a vague recollection of an illustration of the brain in a textbook of Biology which he had seen as a student in seventh standard. However, he maintained that he had never seen a real brain either human or animal, either in museums, exhibitions or at a butcher's shop .... (Rao, 1992)

These conditions all point to severe disruption in the relationship between the self and the body. They can occur in a variety of medical conditions including the following: traumatic brain injury, epilepsy, schizophrenia, migraine, depression, and anxiety. The neural mechanisms underlying autoscopy are still not fully understood. However, research suggests that these phenomena might be related to alterations in the brain's perception and self-awareness networks. Some studies have implicated brain regions such as the temporo-parietal junction, which is involved in spatial perception and body representation, as well as the medial prefrontal cortex, which is associated with self-referential processing. Functional neuroimaging studies have shown abnormal activation patterns in these regions during autoscopy experiences. To further clarify the role of the temporo-parietal junction, it is thought to be a transmodal centre that receives inputs from multiple sensory modalities such as vision, audition, and touch. It also has a role in various cognitive processes such as attention, perception, memory, and social cognition. The temporo-parietal junction helps us to combine information from various sensory modalities so that we can have a coherent and holistic experience of the world.

Additionally, disruptions in the balance between the brain's internal models for self and external reality have been proposed as a potential mechanism. It's important to note that our understanding of autoscopy is still evolving, and further research is needed to fully comprehend the neural basis of this intriguing phenomenon. I will return to these matters in the following chapter. For a fuller discussion, see Oyebode (2021).

These phenomena sit within an age-old dispute within the philosophy of mind and cognitive science, namely the distinction to be made between the dualist theories that derive from Descartes' notions and the monistic theories that refute Cartesian duality. In other words, the question is whether autoscopy, heautoscopy proper, and out-of-the-body experience are clinical and concrete examples of the concept of Cartesian duality, thereby confirming the dual nature of the relationship between the self and the body. This issue points at the importance of autoscopy and related phenomena not only for illuminating the neural underpinning of the representation of the self but also our conceptualization of ourselves as human beings. These matters will be discussed in greater detail later. It is possible that there may be a multiplicity of neural representations of the body that are liable to fracture in given conditions and that the phenomena that are described in this chapter shed some light on these representations.

Dissociative Identity Disorder

Dissociative identity disorder, which was previously known as multiple personality disorder, is a complex psychological condition characterized by the presence of two or more distinct identity states or personalities within an individual. These distinct identities may have their own unique names, mannerisms, memories, and experiences. The person with this condition may experience gaps in memory and lose track of time, commonly referred to as dissociative amnesia. Mitchill (1816) is usually credited with the first description of dissociative identity disorder. The patient was Mary Reynolds, a young English woman, who had emigrated with her family to Pennsylvania. In her early twenties, she is reported to have

> Unexpectedly and without any kind of forewarning, ... [fallen] into a profound sleep, which continued several hours beyond the ordinary term. On waking she was discovered to have lost every trait of acquired knowledge. Her memory was *tabula rasa*; all vestiges of words and things were obliterated and gone. It was found necessary for her to learn everything again ... after a few months another fit of somnolence invaded her. On rousing from it, she found herself restored to the state she was before the paroxysm; but was wholly ignorant of every event and occurrence that had befallen her afterwards ... she is as unconscious of her double character as two distinct persons are of their respective natures ... During, four years upwards, she has undergone periodical transitions from one of these states to the other.

We know that variants of what is now thought of as dissociative personality had been recognized as part of the phenomenon of possession before the nineteenth century. In that period, the experiences attracted a religious overtone, in which two distinct souls were in conflict over control of the subject, and the subject of the experience was aware of the competing forces. In another form of possession, the so-called somnambulistic possession, the subject loses consciousness of his own self while a mysterious intruder appears to take possession of his body and acts and speaks with an individuality of which the subject knows nothing when he returns to awareness. Ellenberger (Figure 7.1), in his magisterial text, *The Discovery of the Unconscious*, explores the evolution of psychological theories and practices related to the concept of the unconscious over time. Ellenberger covers the contributions of Sigmund Freud, Carl Gustav Jung, and, importantly, Pierre Janet whose work in the field of dissociation and the unconscious is important for an understanding of dissociative identity disorder.

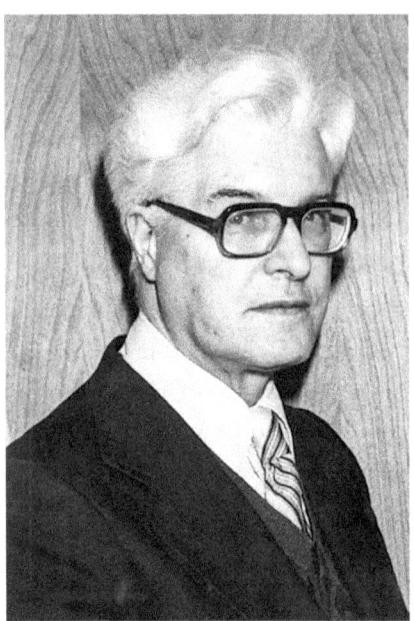

Figure 7.1 Henri Ellenberger 1905–1993. Division des archives et de la gestion de l'information (DAGI) de l'Université de Montréal

Ellenberger makes the point that there are parallels between these two forms of possession and dissociative identity disorder – both can be latent, either occurring under the influence of hypnosis or developing spontaneously (Ellenberger, 1970).

Ellenberger quotes Eberhardt Gmelin's case, published in 1791 as one of the older cases:

> In 1789, at the beginning of the French Revolution, aristocratic refugees arrived in Stuttgart. Impressed by their sight, a twenty-year-old German young woman suddenly 'exchanged' her own personality for the manners and ways of a French-born lady, imitating her and speaking French perfectly and German as would a French woman. These 'French' states repeated themselves. In her French personality, the subject had complete memory of all that she had said and done during her previous French states. As a German, she knew nothing of her French personality. With a motion of his hand, Gmelin was easily able to make her shift from one personality to the other. (Ellenberger, 1981)

The best-known case and one that laid the groundwork for the format of much of the modern cases, providing the model for the structure of the experience, is that by Morton Prince (1906), *The Dissociation of a Personality: A Biographical Study in Abnormal Psychology*, which was published in 1906. Morton wrote:

> Miss Christine L. Beauchamp, the subject of this study, is a person in whom several personalities have become developed; that is to say, she may change personality from time to time, often from hour to hour, and with each change her character becomes transformed and her memories altered. In addition to the real, original or normal self, the self that was born and which she intended by nature to be, she may be any of the three persons. I say three different, because, although making use of the same body, each nevertheless, has distinctly different character: a difference manifested by different trains of thought, by different views, and temperament, and by different acquisitive tastes, habits, experiences, and memories.

Morton Prince's account has become the classic text on dissociative identity disorder. He described multiple personalities/identities embodied in the one person. Morton's account assumed that the body of Miss Beauchamp was incidental to the activities of these personalities, since it was the psychology that determined identity not the readily identifiable and unchanging body.

What we have here is the possibility that multiple or indeed plural identities with their own names, memories, attitudes, and dispositions can inhabit a single body. This possibility challenges any notion of a unified and integrated sense of self over time. The proposition is not merely that there are different aspects, different traits to the one unified individual, but that significant and discrete distinctions of identity can cohabit in the same body.

In the next section, I discuss the delusional misidentification syndrome, conditions that are underpinned by an implicit belief in the possibility, if not the probability, of doubles. The delusions, the false convictions, are organized around the principle that doubles exist and that these doubles can act as impostors either by resembling another person or by masquerading as unknown people.

Delusional Misidentification Syndromes

The term 'delusional misidentification syndromes' refers to a group of relatively rare psychiatric disorders characterized by delusions involving the misidentification or alteration of the identity of oneself or others. There are several types of delusional misidentification syndromes, each with its own distinct characteristics. Some of the notable delusional misidentification syndromes include Capgras syndrome, Frégoli syndrome, delusion of intermetamorphosis, and the delusion of subjective doubles. These conditions are of great and continuing interest to psychiatrists, neuropsychologists, neuroscientists, and philosophers alike because of their intriguing clinical presentations and the fact of the possibility of linking discrete beliefs to neural and neuropsychological underpinnings.

The Capgras syndrome is perhaps one of the best known and most discussed examples of the delusional misidentification syndromes. It is characterized by the firmly held but false belief that an impostor has replaced a familiar person (Capgras, 1923; Silva & Leong, 1992; Ellis et al., 1994; Christodoulou et al., 2009; Abbate et al., 2012).

In Frégoli syndrome, the subject believes that an unfamiliar person is really a disguised familiar person, whereas in the syndrome of intermetamorphosis, the subject believes that the unfamiliar and familiar persons are identical because of shared physical characteristics such as hair colour or shape of nose. The syndrome of subjective doubles is characterized by the belief that a double of the self is abroad in the world acting in such a way as to damage the subject's reputation. The delusion of inanimate doubles refers to the belief that inanimate objects have been duplicated and replaced, whereas reduplicative paramnesia refers to the belief that places have been duplicated.

As I have already discussed, central to these conditions is the concept of the 'double', a concept that was present in mythology and in antiquity and has carried on into fictional narrative and cinema, to the present day. Plautus's *Amphitryon* is a Roman tragicomedy in which Jupiter takes on Amphitryon's appearance in order to sleep with Alcmena, Amphitryon's wife. Mercury takes on Sosia's (Amphitryon's servant) appearance in order to delay Amphitryon's return. The success of this comedy of errors turns on the concept of doubles – Jupiter acting as Amphitryon and Mercury as Sosia. This story was the source of the original name for Capgras syndrome, namely *illusion de Sosie*.

The notion of the double is important in popular culture and as a device in literature and cinema, as already described in Chapter 1, because of the implications regarding the fragility of identity by way of facial recognition and also because of the challenges it posits to our notion of the physical uniqueness of persons, a uniqueness that is only truly in doubt in the case of identical twins. The possibility that persons, objects, places, and even time might not be unique is at the core of delusional misidentification syndromes. This idea that duplication is possible and that against better judgement it can be judged to be self-evident and established even in the face of counterargument and factual impossibility raises a welter of queries, as much about normal processes as about abnormal phenomena. Among the many questions is how we come to recognize faces, people, objects, places, and so on. And how we come to identify them as unique examples of a class of objects, even in the context of marked changes over time. I mean by this the fact that we continue to identify an individual from cradle to grave as the same person, despite significant changes in physiognomy, physique, and facial appearance over time. The fascination with the delusional misidentification syndromes is determined by the many theoretical, philosophical, and empirical matters that they raise. There is the added underlying assumption that these conditions may provide the basis for examining and investigating the neural and pathophysiological basis of delusions in general.

Capgras Syndrome

The Capgras syndrome was first described by French psychiatrists Jean Marie Joseph Capgras and Jean Reboul-Lachaux in 1923. In their case report, Capgras and Reboul-Lachaux presented the details of their patient, a fifty-three-year-old woman referred to as 'Madame M'. She exhibited a peculiar conviction that her husband had been replaced by an imposter who looked and acted like him but was not genuinely him. She said: 'if this person is my husband, he is more than unrecognizable, he is a completely transformed person. I can assure you that the imposter

[sic] husband that they are trying to insinuate as my own husband, has not existed for ten years, is not the person who is keeping me here'. She believed that her children were also objects of substitution. She said: 'they always gave me some other girl, who in turn was taken away and then immediately replaced ... As soon as they took one child away they gave me another who looks just the same: I have had more than two thousand in five years: they are doubles'.

She believed, too, that she was substituted at birth and that her father had acted criminally to abduct and hide her from her real parents, the Duke of Broglie and Mlle de Rio-Branco, the daughter of the Duke of Luynes. She said: 'never having divulged my birth, many people only know the name of the person who brought me up; it's these doubles who have given me the name of their children, that's why they have changed my personal details'. This was a complex case with multiple abnormal beliefs, but the beliefs in doubles were central to her presentation.

Frégoli Syndrome

Frégoli syndrome was first described in 1927 by Courbon and Fail (1927). Their case was a twenty-seven-year-old woman who said that her 'persecutors are capable of all types of transformation and can impose such transformations on others: they are Frégoli who can frégolify any and everybody'. She believed that she was 'the victim of enemies, of whom the main culprits [were] the actresses Robine and Sarah Bernhardt, whom she often went to see in the theatre'. She believed that 'for years they [had] pursued her closely, taking the form of people she knows or meets, taking over her thoughts, preventing her from doing this or that, then forcing her to do things, stroking her and forcing her to masturbate'. She 'recognized members of her own family among the other actors. A female employer who had attempted to caress her three years earlier was Robine. The woman she met and attacked in the street because of the annoying sensation she felt coming from her was also Robine ... The hospital doctor who has never been to Choisy nor bears any resemblance to anyone she has ever known, becomes her dead father or even Dr Leroux, a doctor who saved her when she was three months old, whom she has never seen since and whose features she cannot recall. In the same way, the intern becomes her cousin'.

Frégoli syndrome was aptly named after Leopoldo Frégoli, an Italian actor and quick-change artist who was active in the late nineteenth and early twentieth centuries. He is best known for his remarkable ability to change his appearance and impersonate different characters rapidly during his stage performances. Frégoli's talent earned him the nickname 'The Man with a Thousand Faces'. He would seamlessly switch between costumes and personas in a matter of seconds, creating an illusion of multiple actors on stage. Frégoli's performances were highly entertaining for the audiences of his time.

This condition is dependent on the belief that it is possible to masquerade as others: in this instance, the belief is that an unfamiliar person, a stranger, can actually be a familiar other who is pretending to be a stranger. In other words, a familiar person is doubling as a stranger. The question is, what features the patient is using to determine identity given that physical identity is often very different indeed.

Syndrome of Subjective Doubles

Lastly, syndrome of subjective doubles is a condition that was described by George Christodoulou (1978) in 1978. The patient was an eighteen-year-old woman who believed that a

> female neighbour had succeeded, by means of elaborate transformations, in acquiring physical characteristics identical with her own ("same face, same build, same clothes, same everything"). She believed that this woman had special make-up, a wig, and a mask and characterized this transformation as a "metamorphosis". She later insisted that "she had seen at least two female patients transformed into her own self. She attacked one of these patients and pulled her hair. When her hypothetical double managed to escape from her Ms. A was agonized and begged her doctor to pull the mask" from the other patient's face to disclose her real identity.

She wrote to her father,

> In here there is a girl as fat and as tall as I am. At night when everyone is asleep she puts on a wig and a mask and walks from the room stealing things in order to incriminate me. One night I woke and saw her with my

own eyes. It is unfortunate that due to my confusion I failed to run to the window to shout to the people, "Look here, this is me, and this is my double with a wig and a mask".

The beliefs evident in the syndrome of subjective doubles form the basis of Shusaku Endo's novel, *Shame*. The double acts in the world with the express aim of impugning a person's character and reputation. The belief is not necessarily dependent on seeing the double, but rather it depends on the belief that such a person exists. In the original case, the putative double who is identified with the patient is accused of subterfuge and elaborate transformations to achieve the identical appearance.

Summary

The delusional misidentification syndromes have an influence, quite remarkable, given the relative rarity of the conditions. Their importance lies in their resemblance to a neurological condition, prosopagnosia, which is the impairment of recognizing familiar faces. Given that we know quite a lot about the neurological underpinnings of prosopagnosia, there was hope that the delusional misidentification syndromes would readily yield their underlying pathophysiology and hence that a discrete psychiatric phenomenon will become tractable and understandable. Much progress has been made in our understanding of the fundamental abnormalities in delusional misidentification syndromes, but, nonetheless, there is much yet to understand.

Dissociative identity disorder has a long antiquity and was preceded by possession states, conditions that occur within all human cultures and that are not only found in psychiatric settings. These states point to the capacity for dissociation, a psychological mechanism often associated with childhood traumatic experiences. The underlying mechanisms of both delusional misidentification syndromes and dissociative identity disorder are outside of the scope of this book, but detailed descriptions can be found in *Psychopathology of Rare and Unusual Syndromes* (Oyebode, 2021).

In the following chapter, I will focus on the neural basis and the tentative explanatory hypothesis of autoscopy. It is autoscopy and related conditions that most exemplify what it is to have the experience of a double. In autoscopy, there is not simply a sense of presence but also a visual hallucination of the self, phenomena that are intriguing and astonishing. The use of the double motif in literature and in cinema is not necessarily faithful to the phenomena as seen in the clinic, but, nonetheless, a fuller understanding of the contribution of empirical science to our understanding of autoscopy may also go some way in refining the ways in which fiction and cinema deal with the double motif.

CHAPTER 8

The Double in Neuroscience

That man, sir, is either an impostor – or your twin brother. I've never seen two men more alike; you and him – he and you – water is not more like water nor milk like milk than you two are.

(Titus Maccius Plautus c. 254–c. 184 BC)

The central core feature of autoscopy in all its manifestations is the visual perception, a hallucination, of one's own body in an outside spatial position and usually as a mirror image. In heautoscopy proper, the perception may be anomalous in appearance, with a grey appearance, and the size may be distorted. The perceived body may act autonomously, and, surprisingly, the individual may perceive the world from the perspective of the hallucinatory body. In the circumstance where the autoscopy takes the form of an out-of-the-body experience, the hallucinatory body is usually in an elevated position and the real body lies prone and is seen from the elevated perspective of the hallucinatory body. The popular terms 'the double' and 'doppelgänger' refer to the same phenomena and have a wider reach when used in literature and cinema.

Neuroscience investigations need to explain how it is possible for there to be a visual experience of one's own body in an outside spatial position, in other words, how the double is created. Secondly, there is a need to explain how the double comes to be able to have a viewpoint, a visual perspective, that supplants that of the originating body. To put this phenomenon more clearly, how the double that is merely a hallucinatory body with no material sense organs can come to perceive the world, at all. Finally, given that autoscopy occurs almost exclusively in the context of neurological and psychiatric disorders, what do the lesions responsible for autoscopy tell us about the integration of the self and body, and is it possible to induce normal people to have experiences that are indistinguishable from autoscopy. In the next and final chapter, I will deal with the implications of these empirical inquiries for our concepts of the self and body and how to think of the relationship of self and body.

My starting point is Melzack's (1990) notion of neuromatrix. This notion suggests that the basic experience of our bodies is not merely derived from a sensory pathway with inputs from sensory receptors. Rather, that a network of neurons, a neuromatrix, which consists of loops that integrate the somatosensory thalamus and cortex, the limbic system, and the association cortex, exists a priori, and determines our perception of our bodies. And this perception is dynamic, fluid, and constantly changing depending on our position in the spatial world. To put this in another way, it is not just that we know where our arms and legs are because we receive sensory information from our arms and legs but that there exists an integrated neural circuitry, what Melzack terms a neuromatrix, that is already present from birth and that comes to be influenced by sensory inputs from birth onwards. This model allows us to account for the empirical fact that children with congenitally absent limbs, phocomelia, can and do experience phantom limbs, which shows that our perception of our body is not a passive process that merely reflects inputs from the body but that it is continuously generated by a distributed neural network, the neuromatrix. The neuromatrix is conceived of as having stable genetic determinants and variable spatial and temporal inputs. This means that our body, as an integrated and unified object, has neural representation denoting this unity. This representation reflects all the different sensory inputs including tactile, somatic, proprioceptive, kinaesthetic, visual, and vestibular inputs.

The profound implication of this is that there may be multiple bodily schemas, determined by the different sensory inputs, namely tactile, somatic, proprioceptive, kinaesthetic, visual, and vestibular. These differing inputs, at least theoretically, may be dissociable and thus raise the possibility that our somatic body representation may be dissociable from, say, our proprioceptive body representation. The anomalous bodily experiences seen in the clinics, for instance in autoscopy, whereby the somatic and material body is experienced as separated from the visual/virtual body that is spatially displaced, are pointers to the fundamental fact of multiple sensory inputs and to the possibility of their differentiation. In ordinary day-to-day experience, these differing inputs cohere to form an integrated experience of the self and body.

Olaf Blanke (Figure 8.1), a neurologist and neuroscientist, working with colleagues, has conducted several investigations into the neural and cognitive mechanisms underpinning autoscopy. They show that in cases where focal brain damage is associated with out-of-the-body experience, often there is involvement of either the temporal region or parietal region or both, and there is a suggestion that right-sided lesions predominate. This suggests that autoscopy (autoscopic hallucination and heautoscopy proper) reflects the failure of integration of proprioceptive, tactile, and visual information regarding one's own body, resulting in discrepant representation and ultimately leading to seeing one's own body in a position that does not coincide with the tactile/proprioceptive/

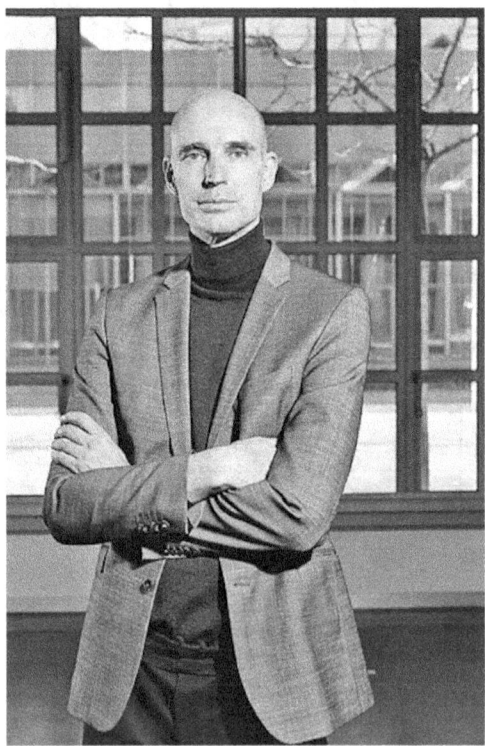

Figure 8.1 Olaf Blanke 1969–present. EPFL, CC 4.0

kinaesthetic experienced position. To simplify this, in autoscopy, the visual self, that is, the visual image of the self, is dissociated from the tactile/proprioceptive/kinaesthetic images, but, importantly, the visuo-spatial perspective is retained as body centred. The virtual, spatially displaced body does not have vision. Impairment or alteration in multi-sensory integration appears at least to contribute to the phenomenon of autoscopy (Blanke and Arzy, 2005). These studies also point to the role of the temporo-parietal junction in encoding for self-location in space and in the ascription of first-person perspective. The evidence comes from studies on patients with epilepsy awaiting surgery in whom stimulation of the angular gyrus results in out-of-the-body experience, and in the use of transcranial magnetic stimulation to the temporo-parietal junction of healthy participants.

Olaf Blanke and colleagues identify three components to out-of-the-body experience, namely disembodiment that is defined as the location of the experiencing self as being outside of one's somatic/material body; an extracorporeal/egocentric perspective that involves seeing the world from a distant and elevated visuo-spatial perspective; and autoscopy that does not involve seeing one's own body from this elevated perspective. They conclude from their review of the neurological literature that in autoscopic phenomena (including autoscopic hallucination and heautoscopy proper), there is no disembodiment, and even where there is disembodiment such as in heautoscopy proper, the self is localized at multiple extracorporeal positions, but the visuo-spatial perspective is always body centred. These clarifications are important because they help us to fully understand the distinction between disembodiment, spatial localization, and visual–spatial perspective. To underline the point, in autoscopy, there is visual hallucination of the self, but no disembodiment, and the visuo-spatial experience is always centred on the material body. Autoscopy can, therefore, be differentiated from out-of-the-body experience by its phenomenology.

In an in-depth study of six subjects, Blanke et al. (2004) definitively show that brain dysfunction in the temporo-parietal junction is associated with out-of-the-body experiences and autoscopy. All cases describing out-of-the-body experiences were characterized by what Blanke and colleagues termed a 'parasomatic' body, that is, a body outside of the physical body. The visuo-spatial experience of this parasomatic body was experienced as immediately elevated and described as inverted by 180 degrees with respect to the extra-personal visual space and their habitual physical body position. In addition, the parasomatic body was 2–3 metres above their actual physical bodies. The experiences were often described as vivid and veridical but sometimes as dreamlike. Self-recognition of the parasomatic body was immediate even when the face was not seen. In all out-of-the-body experiences, the actual physical body was lying prone on the ground or in bed, whereas autoscopic hallucination involved seeing their hallucinated body in an upright standing or sitting position. All patients who experienced out-of-the-body sensations reported vestibular sensations such as feelings of flying or floating.

Blanke and colleagues make a case for the involvement of vestibular mechanisms, particularly graviceptive functions deriving from otoliths that seem to induce sensations of floating and of a sense of elevation in out-of-the-body experiences. The proposition is that otolith dysfunction may have an important causal role in out-of-the-body experience (Blanke and Arzy, 2005). The vestibular dysfunction leads to disembodiment and the elevated visuo-spatial perspective because of the discrepancy between personal (vestibular) space and extra-personal (visual) space.

In the in-depth investigation reported in 2004, Blanke and colleagues find that complex partial epilepsy was the cause of the reported out-of-the-body or autoscopic hallucinatory experience in four of six patients and transitory familial hemiplegic migraine in one patient, and in the sixth patient, the experience was artificially induced by electrical stimulation of the cortex distant from the primary epileptic focus. In conclusion, Blanke et al. (2004) proposed that the main forms of autoscopy (autoscopic hallucination, heautoscopy proper, and out-of-the-body experience) result from a double disintegration in (a) personal space and (b) between personal and extra-personal space at the temporo-parietal junction.

These are complex concepts. Personal space and extra-personal space are two concepts used to describe different spatial zones and boundaries in relation to an individual's body and their surroundings. Personal space refers to the area immediately surrounding an individual's body, typically within arm's length. It is a region that individuals consider as an extension of their personal boundaries. The size of personal space can vary across cultures and individuals, but it generally serves the purpose of protecting one's physical and psychological well-being. Personal space is typically reserved for close friends, family members, and intimate partners, and violation of personal space can lead to feelings of discomfort or intrusion. Blanke suggests that personal space is determined by vestibular mechanisms and underpinned by graviceptive receptors in the otoliths.

On the other hand, extra-personal space refers to the area beyond an individual's personal space, extending into the environment. It refers to the larger physical space that individuals perceive and interact with beyond their immediate vicinity. Extra-personal space encompasses the surrounding environment, including the objects, people, and structures in the distance. It is the space we navigate and interact with in daily life and is determined by visual perception.

The perception and regulation of personal space and extra-personal space involve different cognitive processes and social norms. Personal space tends to be more tightly regulated and influenced by cultural and social factors. It is highly subjective and varies between individuals based on factors such as age, gender, and familiarity with others. Violating personal space without consent can lead to discomfort, anxiety, or a feeling of intrusion. In contrast, extra-personal space is collectively shared and regulated by social and environmental cues. It is influenced by factors such as social norms, architectural design, and societal expectations. For example, people in a crowded city street are aware of maintaining a certain distance from others to avoid collisions, and this distance can vary depending on cultural customs and social context.

In summary, personal space refers to the immediate area around an individual's body, while extra-personal space encompasses the larger physical environment beyond personal boundaries. Personal space is subjective and varies between individuals, while extra-personal space is regulated by social and environmental factors. Both concepts play a role in our daily interactions and navigation of the world around us.

Essentially, Blanke and colleagues argue that there is a requirement of an integration of our representation of our bodies with our representation of extra-personal space for rapid and effective enactment of action within our surroundings. They speculate that ambiguous inputs from proprioceptive, tactile, visual, and vestibular information underlie the anomalous experiences that are described as autoscopy. In further work, Blanke and Mohr (2005) compared patients with autoscopy with those with heautoscopy and showed right hemispheric dominance in patients with out-of-the-body experience and autoscopy, while left hemisphere dominance was demonstrable in patients with heautoscopy. In all three forms of autoscopy, there was involvement of both temporal and parietal lobes. These findings suggest that disembodiment from one's own body is determined by independent mechanisms that are distinct from the mechanisms involved in perspective taking (Cacioppo, 2016).

Finally, in a number of experiments, Blanke and colleagues (Lopez et al., 2008; Lopez & Blanke, 2010; Aspell et al., 2009, 2011; Ionta et al., 2011a, 2011b) show, using robotic technology, that it is possible to induce fundamental changes to the sense of self-location of healthy subjects. These changes were accompanied by demonstrable activity in the temporo-parietal junction using functional magnetic resonance imaging. These experiments confirmed that the temporo-parietal junction encodes self-location and furthermore that multisensory integration at the temporo-parietal junction is responsible for the feeling of being an entity localized at a specific position in space and perceiving the world from this position and perspective. It is beyond the scope of this book to describe in detail these ingenious experiments (see Ionta et al. (2011b) for details). An example of the experimental approach involves participants viewing a three-dimensional video image on a head-mounted display that was linked to a video camera that was placed 2 metres behind the subject, filming the participants from behind. Participants thus saw their body from an 'outside' third-person perspective. In one study using this approach, subjects viewed the video image of their body (the 'virtual body') while an experimenter stroked their back with a stick. The stroking was thus felt by the participants on their backs and seen on the back of the virtual body. The head-mounted display showed the stroking of the virtual body either in real time or not, therefore generating synchronous and asynchronous visuo-tactile stimulation (Blanke, 2012).

These ingenious and elegant experiments demonstrate that subjects who viewed the video image of their body while an experimenter stroked their back with a stick experienced illusory self-identification with the virtual body, and referral of touch to the virtual body was stronger during synchronous rather than asynchronous stroking. Taking account of the different approaches used to keep motor and vestibular factors constant while investigating visuo-tactile stimulation, the authors were able to show that a subject could experience tactile sensation located in a virtual body, and, in addition, this illusory self-identification with the virtual body includes nociceptive and physiological changes such as skin conductance response to a threat directed towards the virtual body (Blanke, 2012).

Furthermore, Blanke (2012) shows that egocentric versus allocentric mental transformations have distinct brain processes. In this context, the term allocentric refers to a perspective or frame of reference that is centred on external objects or landmarks, rather than oneself. It is commonly used in psychology and cognitive science to describe the way individuals perceive and navigate their environment. An allocentric perspective involves understanding and processing spatial information in relation to things outside of oneself, such as landmarks, other objects, or the surrounding environment. In contrast, an egocentric perspective relates to understanding and perceiving the environment relative to oneself.

In Blanke's study, when participants are asked to imagine shifting their position and perspective to a new position and perspective in space and make judgements about variable attributes or spatial relations of stimuli from the imagined position and perspective, these mental operations are associated with activation in the right middle temporal gyrus, supplementary motor area, left middle occipital gyrus and in the left temporo-parietal junction. When subjects are asked to generate egocentric mental imagery by imagining themselves at the position and perspective of virtually presented human figures, there is associated activation of bilateral temporo-parietal junction and bilateral extrastriate cortex in proximity to the extrastriate body area. Allocentric mental transformations are associated with activation of the right posterior parietal cortex.

The role of the vestibular-related areas has been studied by exposure of healthy subjects to weightlessness, caloric, and galvanic stimulation of the inner ear with the consequence of disintegration of bodily information and altered body ownership and embodiment, thereby further clarifying the contributions of the vestibular processing to these issues (Lopez et al., 2008).

These hypotheses linking the temporo-parietal junction to autoscopy were confirmed in a report of a patient who experienced out-of-the-body experience during an awake craniotomy for resection for a low-grade glioma. Stimulation of the subcortical white matter in the left temporo-parietal junction repetitively induced out-of-the-body experiences. The patient described floating above the operating table and looking down on herself (Bos et al., 2016). In a different report, two patients with epilepsy had electrical stimulation of the right medial occipitoparietal cortex including the right precuneus and occipitoparietal sulcus and reported seeing their own faces, facing themselves in the left visual field. This study suggests that the stimulated region may be involved in representations of our own face (Jonas et al., 2014). Nakul and Lopez (2017) make the point that out-of-the-body experience is very rarely induced by electrical brain stimulation, and they conclude, from this, that it suggests that neural underpinnings of the anchoring of the self to the body must be exceedingly robust and that in the case reported by Bos et al., the effect was produced by stimulation of subcortical tracts. Indirect confirmation for the role of the temporo-parietal junction was reported by the finding in another study in a patient who had electro-encephalograph recordings during heautoscopy experience and a right parietal electrical focus (Anzellotti et al., 2011).

In summary, Blanke and his colleagues have made significant contributions to our understanding of autoscopy and out-of-the-body experiences. Their research has shed light on the neural and cognitive mechanisms underlying these experiences. By employing techniques such as electrical stimulation, virtual reality, and transcranial magnetic stimulation, they have uncovered the involvement of brain regions like the angular gyrus and temporo-parietal junction in the generation of autoscopy. Furthermore, their work has emphasized the role of multisensory integration, visual-motor coordination, and psychological factors in the manifestation of these experiences. These findings have advanced our knowledge of the complex nature of autoscopy and its implications for our understanding of self-consciousness and bodily perception and reminded us, too, that healthy subjects are susceptible to these experiences in the context of experimental conditions.

Summary

Autoscopy is an important clinical condition because it sits, very precisely, at the centre of an age-long debate about the nature of the mind–body relationship. The reported clinical experiences suggest, at the very least, that it is possible for there to be a visual doppelgänger, a double of one's own body or, at the most extreme, in out-of-the-body experiences that this doppelgänger, the so-called parasomatic body, can have a visual experience from its elevated position and perspective. In other words, a virtual self without sensory organs can perceive the world from its perspective.

Philosophical discussions about the nature of the mind–body relationship rarely, if ever, consider the empirical literature from autoscopy. In the following chapter, I explore what implications autoscopy has for our notions of the self and its relationship with the body.

CHAPTER 9

The Ultimate Illusion

Understanding Embodiment and the Self

I possess a body with which I am very intimately conjoined, yet because, on the one side, I have a clear and distinct idea of myself inasmuch as I am only a thinking and unextended thing, and as, on the other hand, I possess a distinct idea of body, inasmuch as it is only an extended and unthinking thing, it is certain that this I (that is to say, my soul by which I am what I am), is entirely and absolutely distinct from my body, and can exist without.

(René Descartes 1569–1650)

The focus of this book is the extent to which the double motif, the idea of the doppelgänger, pervades mythology, folklore, fiction, and cinema. And also how this motif is itself grounded, at least to some extent, in psychopathology and neuroscience. There is persisting and enduring preoccupation with the double motif in human popular culture. This preoccupation explores both the double as other and as duality.

There is little doubt that René Descartes's (1596–1650) dualism is partly responsible for the interest in the double motif. His thesis, that we are ultimately thinking beings that are distinct from our bodies and that are capable of existing without our bodies, underpins much of the flourishing of notions of the double as other and as duality. There are insurmountable difficulties for classical Cartesian dualism, not least the unexplained but obvious fact of how the two distinct substances, mind and body, could possibly interact to produce the integrated unity of experience that everyone is subjectively aware of.

Nonetheless, there are persisting and outstanding issues that, on the face of it, seem intractable for an argument that says that there is only one substance, the physical and material body and brain. And that mental states just are instantiated in this material substance. To exemplify this point, the subjective experience of pain, that is, what it feels like to be in pain, is different in kind from a materialist description of how pain is caused. In other words, the subjective experience of pain is irreducible to a materialist account (see Nagel, 1995). To emphasize this point, the claim is that a materialist account cannot exhaust all that there is to say about my personal subjective experience of pain or of any mental event for that matter.

The account that follows, of how our sense of self is created, can be regarded as a materialist description as it locates the experience of the self in particular brain structures and then seeks to explain how the experience of a doppelgänger can be accommodated within a materialist account given the superficial resemblance to what one might expect in the light of classical Cartesian dualism.

As a preamble, it is worth noting that a materialist theory that advocates the identification of mental states and events with physical processes in the brain can be termed an identity theory (Kim, 1996). Thus, certain anatomical and physiological configurations and processes of the brain make the experiencing of the self possible. Jaegwon Kim's (1996) ultimate goal is to replace mentalistic language with physical language; once mental states are systematically identified with neural correlates, for as he says, this will facilitate conceptual and linguistic simplicity. That is not the aim of this book. My goal is to turn our attention to what we know about the neurological underpinnings of the experiencing of the self in the normal everyday mode and genuinely intriguing subjective experience of doppelgänger phenomenon.

There are two varieties of identity theories: type identity theory and token identity theory. For a fuller explication of these theories, see McGinn (1997). Neither of these theories on their own go anywhere near being adequate to capture the facts of the empirical findings about the relationship between mental states and their neural correlates. Type identity theory, for example, attempts to give a materialist account that allows us to both identify mental properties with physical properties while also allowing room for the distinctive features of mental states such as subjectivity by keeping mental and physical concepts separate. Token identity theory, on the other hand, argues that every mental event is identical with some physical event, although the properties by virtue of which an event is mental are not themselves physical properties

(McGinn, 1997). This approach is problematic precisely because it makes no commitment to mind body reduction. Yet, we know from the empirical literature that there are intimate connections and relations between the mental and the physical. As I go on to demonstrate, the relations between the mental and the physical are not arbitrary.

The neuroscience project is to develop a detailed understanding and explanation of the relation between the mental and physical. This project requires the mapping of our naïve views about our mental states, namely our subjective accounts that largely depend upon introspection to the underlying neural substrate. And it is self-evident that views and judgements based on introspection are liable to error and misunderstanding. This is another way of saying that our common-sense psychological frameworks can be misleading, and the conceptualizations derived from this approach as the basis of theorizing about the causes of human behaviour and about the nature of cognitive activity may not be reliable (Churchland, 1990). This fact does not mean, as Churchland supposes, that psychological language and the notion of mind can be easily eliminated from day-to-day discourse such as they propose in their theory of eliminative materialism. It is true that for our normal encounters with other people, common-sense psychological terms suffice. Furthermore, the neuroscience project requires a degree of correspondence and consistency between our theories of mental events and their physiological causes. It may turn out that our everyday language commits us to a view about mental life, which is at odds with the empirical facts.

Paul Schilder (1886–1940)

I want now to explore Paul Schilder's contributions to our understanding of how the body and self are a synthetic unity. In his book *The Image and Appearance of the Human Body* (Schilder, 1936), he examines the concept of embodiment and the complex relationship between our physical bodies and our sense of self. In this book, Schilder investigates the psychological, sociocultural, and philosophical aspects of body perception and its significance in human experience. At its core, Schilder's work emphasizes that our perception of our body is not limited to its physical attributes, but also includes a subjective, psychological construct that he calls the 'body image'. The body image is the mental representation we have of our own body, including its form, size, and functionality. For Schilder, the image of our body is the picture that we have of our own body in our mind and it is built up from sensations, including visual, tactile, thermal, and pain sensations and incorporating sensations from our muscles and viscera. Schilder argues that our body image is dynamic and fluid, influenced by internal factors such as emotions, sensations, and thoughts, as well as external factors like cultural norms and social interactions.

Schilder distinguishes between body image and body schema. He argues that there is a unity of the body manifest as the body schema and that it is this schema that makes it possible to determine the current position or locality of the body as it is the template on which changes are compared. Otherwise, the constant shifts in posture and position would be impossible to accurately decipher.

Schilder highlights that the body image is not a fixed entity, but rather a malleable construct that develops through a continuous interplay between sensory perceptions and psychological processes. He examines the impact of various psychological factors such as body schema, and body consciousness, on our body image formation. Body schema refers to the internal representation of the body's dimensions and sensory experiences. The distinction between body image and body schema is often glossed over, and the two terms are either conflated or treated as synonyms. Nonetheless, there is a subtle difference between them that is worth keeping in mind.

Moreover, Schilder explores the social and cultural dimensions of the body image. He argues that societal norms, values, and expectations significantly shape our perception of ourselves and our bodies. Cultural factors, such as beauty standards and gender roles, influence how we view and experience our bodies. Schilder emphasizes that these external influences interact with our individual experiences and subjective interpretations to form our unique body image.

Schilder makes the point that his intention is to study the mechanisms by which the central nervous system builds up the spatial image of the body. One of Schilder's most significant postulations was to draw on Sir Henry Head's (1861–1940) original work on the role of the sense of posture in determining our knowledge of our bodies. This is connected, in Schilder's view, with the ability to develop an understanding of the knowledge of the relationship of different parts of the surface of the body to one another. Schilder makes the point that there is an optic (visual) image of the body, which is independent of tactile images. Here we have the beginning of a notion that the body image is a composite of proprioceptive (postural), visual, tactile, and other images. More importantly, these varying perceptual images can be dissociated from one another (see Chapter 8).

Schilder examines the problem of phantom limbs in amputees and concludes that this is an example of the dissociation of the postural image from the visual image: the postural image persists in the absence of the visual image. It could be argued that this is the commonest example of the presence of a virtual body in the absence of a real and material body. Phantom limbs expose the fact that the body image is composed of a variety of underlying sensory images.

Furthermore, there is evidence of continuing participation in motor activity in, for example, the demonstrable presence of associated movements of the phantom. Schilder reports that movement of the left arm provoked a clenching of the fist on the phantom of the right side. The reverse is also true; movement of the phantom limb provokes associated movements in the healthy leg and arm.

What Schilder's cases and writings do is to confirm that virtual bodies exist, and these are revealed, prominently, in amputees with phantom limbs. These virtual bodies are inextricably linked to the central nervous system or, to put it in another way, are only comprehensible given what we know about how the central nervous system generates the body image. There is nothing to suggest that these virtual bodies are independent of the material body.

Antonio Damasio

Antonio Damasio (2011) (Figure 9.1) in his book *Self Comes to Mind* addresses many of the same issues as Schilder but in a modern way, taking account of up-to-date empirical findings in the neurosciences. He makes the point that neuronal networks map the body, thereby constituting

THE ULTIMATE ILLUSION

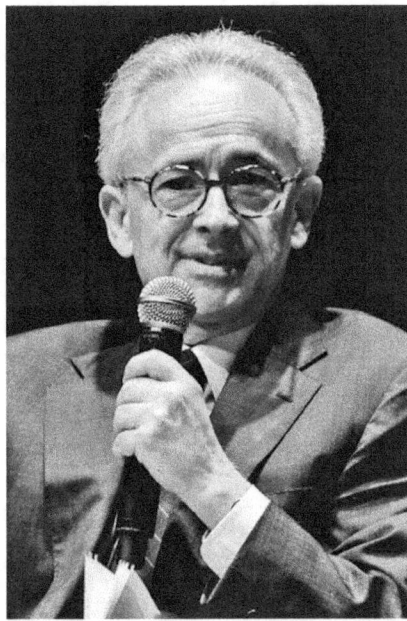

Figure 9.1 Antonio Damasio 1944–present. Fronteiras do Pensamento, CC BY-SA 2.0

a kind of *neural double* of the body. This approach allows us to start to appreciate how the virtual body is created and how even in the absence of parts of the material body, as in an amputee, the neural double remains intact, at least for a period, producing the experience of the phantom limb.

We can begin to glimpse how the brain, as a cartographer, maps the objective world, including the body proper, from the skin through to the muscles and the viscera, and in doing this represents or models in a continuous manner the material body. Damasio exemplifies the mapping capacity of the brain by examining how the eyes come to represent the world outside. What is important here is the way in which the specific pattern of light that strikes the retina is preserved, as in a map, as the transduced neural pattern travels along the optic pathway to the visual cortex. In other words, the geometric relationships of the patterns of parts of the external objects are preserved in the visual cortex. This mapping function of the brain is fundamental to how the brain manages, controls, and preserves life processes. One of Damasio's most important insights was to recognize that feelings too are mapped. In Chapter 8, I have drawn attention to the fact that the representations of the body include varied perceptions including visual, proprioceptive, tactile, and other sensory modalities. Damasio adds to this array a large range of emotional responses such as laughter, crying, disgust, and fear that originate from the periaqueductal grey matter and that are mapped in a complex way. It is difficult to envisage how this map is constructed in comparison to the map of the external visual world. The coordinates and geographical structure of the external visual world are easily comprehensible as they merely mimic how the external world is given to us. On the other hand, emotional responses seem more nebulous, less tractable, than representations of the visual world, for example. Nonetheless, maps of our emotional responses must exist even if they are not constructed in a topographical manner. In order to motivate or discourage behaviour, our attentional fields must be primed by background emotional value that determines what we look out for, what we seek to avoid, and so on.

It is remarkable, if not extraordinary, that the superior colliculus, a structure recognized as being involved in the construction of the visual world, also has topographical maps of auditory and somatic information. These maps are stacked in a precise spatial register that corresponds, allowing for an integration of these disparate maps.

So far, I have been making the case that virtual bodies exist and that these virtual bodies are the result of the brain's role in mapping our material bodies in the same way that it maps the external world. These maps or models of our bodies are dynamic and continually adapting to the realities of our material bodies. These maps are not independent of our bodies, and it is an error to regard the maps as more fundamentally us. In other words, the assertion that we are 'thinking and unextended' things that are distinct from and independent of our bodies is a misunderstanding of the relationship of the body to the self. In fact, even the notion of a material body and its associated virtual body still errs as it seeks to distinguish between the two, as if such a distinction were possible at all.

There is an inextricable unity between the body and the virtual self, and this tight link is the subject of the science of embodiment. Gibbs Jr (2005) in *Embodiment and Cognitive Science* makes the point that how we conceive of ourselves as persons is linked to tactile-kinesthetic activity. In this way, embodiment is more than physiological and/or brain activity, and is constituted by recurring patterns of kinesthetic, proprioceptive actions that provide much of people's felt, subjective experience. The aim here is to provide an explanation for firstly the fact that we are not composed of two kinds of things but rather are a unity, but that, secondly, we experience ourselves as if we were a self in a body. For Gibbs, a body is not just something that we own; it is something that we are. His claim is that the regularities in people's kinesthetic-tactile experience not only constitute the core of their self-conceptions as persons but form the foundation for higher-order cognition.

Gibbs argues that what distinguishes human beings from other animals is the capacity for a first-person perspective, one that allows a person to both conceive of his body and his mental states as being his own. But there is a problem here, in that language itself acts to accentuate the illusion of a separation between self and body in such utterances as 'I have a body'. These kinds of utterances, at least superficially, underscore the separation of the self and the body. Gibbs counters this potential error by making clear that a body is not just something that *we own*, but it is something that *we are* and that, most significantly, there is no self without a body.

In Gibbs's model, our sense of ourselves, as persons, comes from how sensory information is correlated with experience. For example, we know who we are, in part, because we see our bodies (e.g., hands, legs, arms, stomach, feet) as we move and experience specific sensations because of action. The importance of action as a foundational principle in determining our sense of self has not been properly understood in comparison to the role of sensory perception as described in Chapter 8. Our self-concepts depend, at least in part, on the patterns of bodily actions we engage in on. Gibbs puts it this way:

> The sense of agency, as the causal basis for action, is perhaps the most convincing evidence for the 'I' we experience as persons. For instance, I make a conscious decision to raise my right hand, and my body somehow responds accordingly. Much of the persistent belief that we are the 'authors' of our actions is rooted in the systematic patterns of actions that appear to follow from our willful intentions. (pp. 347–349)

Even more profound is the understanding, for example, that the function of vision is not to produce inner experiences or representations, as such, but rather to keep the perceiver in touch with his environment and to guide action. To see an object is already to be prompted to recognize what the object is for and coupled with this is preparing the whole body for action. There is therefore a coalition of perception, meaning, and action. To emphasize this point, Merleau-Ponty's (1962) account of perception in his classic text *Phenomenology of Perception* makes a similar point, namely that perception is irreducible to sensations and that the subject of perception is not a mere spectator, and that perception is not a spectacle. Objects of perception already have value and significance by being perceived. Any object that is seen or heard is given directly and full of meaning and relevance. All perception of the external world is already a component part of our identity as subjects of experience and, more forcefully, is incorporated into the underlying neural representation of our bodies, which is itself constitutive of our selves.

Moheb Costandi

This book is about the nature and narratives of the double – a subject that has preoccupied writers, philosophers, and cognitive scientists to the present day. The enduring interest attests to the compelling nature of the possibility that we are indeed composed of two parts that are distinct in quality and that, on the face of it, are potentially independent of one another. But the empirical evidence leans much more in the direction that the brain creates a virtual self alongside the material body, exactly as it creates a map of the external world, which allows us to successfully negotiate the world that we inhabit. It is this process, the creation of a virtual self composed of several distinct representations of the body, that produces the illusion of a self that is distinct and separable from the body. Moheb Costandi (2022) in *The New Science of Self-consciousness: Body Am I* wrote: 'The brain contains multiple representations of the body, which are crucial for both action and perception, but it is unclear how different bodily representations interact with one another, or exactly how they relate to conscious awareness of the body' (p. 63). Nonetheless, it is now clear that the brain does not perceive the world as it is, but rather that our perception of the world is a model of the external world predicated on the best approximation given the limited information that our senses receive. To put it more strongly, our knowledge of the world is determined by a guess, built on a predictive model, a statistical approximation of the inputs from our senses. What is remarkable is that the self-same processes are involved in how we perceive our bodies. Again, Costandi puts it this way:

> To a large extent, we perceive our body in the same way that we perceive an object in the outside world, through multiple channels of sensory information that enter our brain: the sight of our body as it moves, the sounds it makes, the touch and pain signals that arise from our skin, our muscle sense, and our internal sensations. Our brain integrates all of this information to generate models of our body and the space surrounding it. (Costandi, 2022, p. 166)

What has yet to be fully recognized is the degree to which this brain process, the neural construction of the body, of the virtual self, is the ultimate illusion. A self-consciousness that has the characteristics of a distinct self, an entity that has the subjective experience of selfhood, that seems to be different and distinct from the body. This construction has all the formal characteristics associated with the self: a unique identity that is unified across time, that is an agent of action and that has boundaries that distinguish it from other selves and other objects, and finally that has a sense of vitality, which is of being alive.

This ultimate illusion is accentuated and intensified by language. The word 'I' gives the sense that this self has a reality quite distinct from the reality of the body. It possesses the body by referring to the body as 'my body' and is able to utter sentences such as 'I have a body', all of which perpetuate the illusion that the self and body are separate and separable. But more importantly that the self is superordinate to the body. It is not merely that the body belongs to the self but that the self determines what the body does, that it initiates action, that it gives reasons for action, and that the body is no more than a temple, a house for the self. This is the degree to which this ultimate illusion has a compelling control over the narrative of the relationship between self and body.

It could be argued that folklore narratives and fictional and cinematic narratives are extensions of this innate and compelling ultimate illusion of the manner in which the self relates to the body. On the basis of this conclusion, we ought to and do see literary accounts that explore the possibility of identity not being instantiated in the body; in multiple identities cohabiting in a single body; in a complete severance between the self and the body demonstrating that the body is no more than a convenient house; in the possibility that the self can act upon other bodies, thereby having agency over other bodies; and that the boundaries of the self and other bodies and materials can be melded.

It is surprising that one of the most basic understandings of how the self is constructed, namely, that it is a composite of different perceptual modalities such as proprioception, vision, touch, and somatic perception, and so on, has yet to influence fictional and cinematic narratives. The double in fiction and cinema is invariably visual, rarely ever is it proprioceptive, tactile, or whatever else. Perhaps the imaginative possibilities of a dissociated singularly tactile double or a floating but non-visual double are profoundly difficult to realize and appropriate for art.

Summary

In conclusion, the doppelgänger and the double motifs are basic themes in popular culture. I have argued that they are both based upon phenomena that are well represented in clinical psychopathology and demonstrable in cognitive neuroscience. These are intriguing concepts and experiences that make for wonderful literature and cinema. I have explored how the doppelgänger motif is employed and deployed in classical drama, Greco-Roman theatre, fiction, and cinema, showing the richness and multivaried ways that the motif has developed and been deployed over time and across culture. The influence of these concepts and experiences on popular culture is likely to continue well into the future. However, the empirical literature leads well away from the pervasive and influential Cartesian dualism that seems entrenched in our thinking and that structures our thinking about the relationship of the body to the self. As I have shown, the body, the innervation of the body to be specific, has systems for representing differing sensory aspects of our body. These representations can produce the illusory experience of a doppelgänger under particular conditions, what I term the ultimate illusion. It is this illusion that creates the superficial experience of the double, but as we have seen, this experience is intimately linked to the body and is impossible without the body.

References

Abbate, C., Trimarchi, P. D., Salvi, G. P. et al. (2012). Delusion of inanimate doubles: Description of a case of focal retrograde amnesia. *Neurocase*, 18(6), 457–477.

Anzellotti, F., Onofrj, V., Maruotti, V. et al. (2011). Autoscopic phenomena: Case report and review of literature. *Behavioral and Brain Function*, https://doi.org/10.1186/1744-9081-7-2.

Aspell, J. E., Lenggenhager, B., & Blanke, O. (2009). Keeping in touch with one's self: multisensory mechanisms of self-consciousness. *PloS One*. https://doi.org/10.1371/journal.pone.0006488.

Aspell, J. E., Lenggenhager, B., & Blanke, O. (2011). Multisensory perception and bodily self-consciousness: From out-of body to inside-body experience. https://infoscience.epfl.ch/handle/20.500.14299/57415.

Blanke, O. (2012). Multisensory brain mechanisms of bodily self-consciousness. *Nature Reviews Neuroscience*, 13, 556–571.

Blanke, O, & Arzy, S. (2005). The out-of-body experience: disturbed self-processing at the temporo-parietal junction. *The Neuroscientist*, 11(1). https://doi.org/10.1177/1073858404270885.

Blanke, O., Landis, T., Spinelli, L., & Seeck, M. (2004). Out-of-body experience and autoscopy of neurological origin. *Brain*, 127(2), 243–258.

Blanke, O., & Mohr, C. (2005). Out-of-body experience, heautoscopy, and autoscopic hallucination of neurological origin: Implications for neurocognitive mechanisms of corporeal awareness and self-consciousness. *Brain Research Reviews*, 50(1), 184–199.

Borges, J. L. (1964). *Labyrinths: Selected Stories & Other Writings*. London, Penguin Books.

Borges, J. L. (1977). *The Book of Sand*. London, Penguin Books.

Bos, E. M., Spoor, J. K. H., Smits, M. et al. (2016). Out-of-body experience during awake craniotomy. *World Neurosurgery*, 92, 586.e9–586.e13.

Bradbury, R. (2001). *The Martian Chronicles*. London, Harper Voyager.

Brugger, P., Regard, M., & Landis, T. (1997). Illusory reduplication of one's own body: Phenomenology and classification of autoscopic phenomena. *Cognitive Neuropsychiatry*, 2, 19–38.

REFERENCES

Cacioppo, S. (2016). What happens in your brain during mental dissociation? A quest towards neural markers of a unified sense of self. *Current Behavioral Neuroscience Reports*, 3, 1–9.
Capgras, J. (1923). L'illusion des sosies dans un delire systematique chronique. *Bulletin de la Société Clinique de Médecine Mentale*, 2, 6–16.
Christodoulou, G. N. (1978). Course and prognosis of the syndrome of doubles. *The Journal of Nervous and Mental Disease*, 166(1), 68–72.
Christodoulou, G. N., Margariti, M., Kontaxakis, V. P., & Christodoulou, N. G. (2009). The delusional misidentification syndromes: Strange, fascinating, and instructive. *Current Psychiatry Reports*, 11(3), 185–189.
Churchland, P. M. (1990). *Matter and Consciousness*. Cambridge, MA, MIT Press.
Costandi, M. (2022). *Body Am I: The New Science of Self-Consciousness*. Cambridge: MIT Press.
Courbon, P., & Fail, G. (1927). Syndrome d'illusion de Frégoli et schizophrénie. *Bulletin de la Société Clinique de Médecine Mentale*, 20, 121–125.
Damasio, A. (2011). *Self Comes to Mind: Constructing the Conscious Brain*. London, Random House.
Dostoevskij, F. M., Dostoyevsky, F., & MacAndrew, A. R. (1987). *Selected Letters of Fyodor Dostoyevsky*. New Brunswick, Rutgers University Press.
Dostoyevsky, F. (1846). *The Double* (translated R. Wilks). London, Penguin Books.
Dostoyevsky, F. (2008). *Demons*. London, Penguin UK.
Dostoyevsky, F. (2018). *The Insulted and the Injured* (translated C. Garnett). Toronto: Aegitas.
Eiríksson, L. (1997). Eirik the Red's Saga (translated K. Kunz). In *The Sagas of Icelanders: A selection* (ed. Ö. Thorsson). New York, Viking Penguin.
Ellenberger, H. F. (1970). *The Discovery of the Unconscious*. New York City: Basic Books.
Ellis, B. E. (2005). *Lunar Park*. London, Picador.
Ellis, H. D., Luauté, J. P., & Retterstøl, N. (1994). Delusional misidentification syndromes. *Psychopathology*, 27(3–5), 117–120.
Endō, S. (1988). *Scandal* (translated Van C. Gessel). London, Penguin Books.
Euripides. (1954). *The Bacchae and Other Plays*. London, Penguin Classics.
George, A. (1999). *The Epic of Gilgamesh: A New Translation*. London, Penguin Books.
Gibbs Jr, R. W. (2005). *Embodiment and Cognitive Science*. Cambridge, Cambridge University Press.
Gogol, N. V. (1972). *Diary of a Madman, and Other Stories*. London, Penguin Classics.
Halloran, W. F. (2022). *William Sharp and 'Fiona Macleod': A Life*. Cambridge, Open Book Publishers.
Hoffmann, E. T. A. (2009). *The Devil's Elixirs* (translated R. Taylor). London, One World Classics.
Hogg, J. (2010). *The Private Memoirs and Confessions of a Justified Sinner*. Oxford, Oxford University Press.
Hume, D., & Selby-Bigge, L. A. (1789). *A Treatise of Human Nature*, 3 volumes. Oxford, The Clarendon Press.
Ionta, S., Gassert, R., & Blanke, O. (2011a). Multi-sensory and sensorimotor foundation of bodily self-consciousness–an interdisciplinary approach. *Frontiers in Psychology*. https://doi.org/10.3389/fpsyg.2011.00383.

REFERENCES

Ionta, S., Heydrich, L., Lenggenhager, B. et al. (2011b). Multisensory mechanisms in temporo-parietal cortex support self-location and first-person perspective. *Neuron*, 70(2), 363–374.

Jonas, J., Maillard, L., Frismand, S. et al. (2014). Self-face hallucination evoked by electrical stimulation of the human brain. *Neurology*, 83(4), 336–338. https://doi.org/10.1212/WNL.0000000000000628.

King, S. (1989). *The Dark Half*. New York, Viking Penguin Books.

Kim, J. (1996). *Philosophy of Mind*. Colorado, Westview Press.

Lem, S. (1987). *Solaris*. Boston, Mariner Books.

Lhermitte, J. (1951). Visual hallucination of the self. *British Medical Journal*, 1(4704), 431–434.

Lloyd, C. (2020). *Guy de Maupassant*. London, Reaktion Books.

Lopez, C., & Blanke, O. (2010). How body position influences the perception and conscious experience of corporeal and extrapersonal space. *Revue de neuropsychologie*, 2, 195–202.

Lopez, C., Halje, P., & Blanke, O. (2008). Body ownership and embodiment: Vestibular and multisensory mechanisms. *Neurophysiologie Clinique/Clinical Neurophysiology*, 38(3), 149–161.

Lukianowicz, N. (1967). 'Body image' disturbances in psychiatric disorders. *The British Journal of Psychiatry*, 113(494), 31–47.

Lunn, V. (1970). Autoscopic phenomena. *Acta Psychiatrica Scandinavica*, 46(s219), 118–125. https://doi.org/10.1111/j.1600-0447.1970.tb07987.x.

Maupassant, G. D. (2004). *A Parisian Affair and Other Stories: Trans. Sian Miles*. London, Penguin Books.

McConnell, W. B. (1965). The phantom double in pregnancy. *The British Journal of Psychiatry*, 111(470), 67–69.

McGinn, C. (1997). *The Character of Mind*. 2nd ed. Oxford, Oxford University Press.

McGrath, P. (1990). *Spider*. London, Penguin Books.

Meehan, P. (2017). *The Ghost of One's Self: Doppelgangers in Mystery, Horror and Science Fiction Films*. Jefferson, North Carolina, McFarland.

Melzack, R. (1990). Phantom limbs and the concept of a neuromatrix. *Trends in Neurosciences*, 13(3), 88–92.

Melzack, R., Israel, R., Lacroix, R., & Schultz, G. (1997). Phantom limbs in people with congenital limb deficiency or amputation in early childhood. *Brain*, 120(9), 1603–1620.

Merleau-Ponty, M. (1962). *Phenomenology of Perception* (translated C. Smith). London, Routledge.

Miller, K. (1987). *Doubles: Studies in Literary History*. Oxford, Oxford University Press.

Mitchill, S. L. (1816). A double consciousness, or a duality of person in the same individual. *Medical Repository*, 3, 185–186.

Moravia, S. (1995). *The Enigma of the Mind: The Mind-Body Problem in Contemporary Thought*. Cambridge, Cambridge University Press.

Nabokov, V. V. (1966). *Despair*. London, Penguin Books.

Nagel, T. (1995). *Other Minds: Critical Essays*. Oxford, Oxford University Press.

REFERENCES

Nakul, E., & Lopez, C. (2017). Commentary: Out-of-body experience during awake craniotomy. *Frontiers in Human Neuroscience.* 11, https://doi.org/10.33 89/fnhum.2017.00417.

Oyebode, F. (2021). *Psychopathology of Rare and Unusual Syndromes.* Cambridge, Cambridge University Press.

Plautus, T. M. (1995). *Plautus: The Comedies Volume 1.* Baltimore, The Johns Hopkins University Press.

Plautus, T. M. (2004). *The Pot of Gold and Other Plays* (translated E. T. A. Watling). London, Penguin UK.

Prince, M. (1906). *The Dissociation of a Personality: The Hunt for the Real Miss Beauchamp.* Oxford, Oxford University Press.

Rao, K. N. (1992). Internal autoscopy: A case report. *Indian Journal of Psychiatry,* 34(3), 280–282.

Richter, J. P. R. (1863). *Siebenkäs.* Boston, Ticknor and Fields.

Rogers, R. (1970). *A Psychoanalytic Study of the Double in Literature.* Detroit, Wayne State University Press.

Ryle, G. (1949). *The Concept of Mind.* London, Penguin.

Ryle, G. (1990). *The Concept of Mind.* London, Routledge.

Saramago, J. (2005). *The Double* (translated M. J. Costa). London, Random House.

Schilder, P. (1936). *The Image and Appearance of the Human Body: Studies in the Constructive Energies of the Psyche.* London, Routledge.

Silva, J. A., & Leong, G. B. (1992). The Capgras syndrome in paranoid schizophrenia. *Psychopathology,* 25(3), 147–153.

Smiley, J. (2005). *The Sagas of the Icelanders.* London, Penguin UK.

Spoto, D. (1984). *The Dark Side of Genius: The Life of Alfred Hitchcock.* London, Frederick Muller.

Stevenson, R. L., & Middleton, T. (1993). *Dr Jekyll and Mr Hyde with the Merry Men and Other Stories.* Ware, Hertfordshire, Wordsworth Editions.

Strawson, G. (1997). The self. *Journal of Consciousness Studies,* 4(5–6), 405–428.

Unger, P. (1990). *Identity, Consciousness and Value.* Oxford: Oxford University Press.

Wilkes, K. V., & Wilkes, K. (1988). *Real People: Personal Identity without Thought Experiments.* Oxford, Clarendon Press.

Wilson, R. (2015). *The Man Who Was Jekyll and Hyde: The Lives and Crimes of Deacon Brodie.* Stroud, The History Press.

Index

The 39 Steps (Hitchcock), 106

Aeschylus, 18
agency, Gibbs on the sense of, 159
agnosia, 60
Alcestis (Euripides), 19
allocentric mental transformations, vs. egocentric, 149
alter ego, 4
   in Cameron's *Avatar*, 125
   in Ellis's *Lunar Park*, 75
   in Hitchcock's *Psycho*, 116
   in Hitchcock's *Vertigo*, 114
   in King's *Dark Half*, 72
   in R. L. Stevenson's *Jekyll and Hyde*, 79–80
American Psycho (Ellis), 74, 75
Amphitryron (Plautus), 23–26
   doubles appearing on stage, 23
   mistaken identity in, 24–25, 136
   twin motif in, 24
ancient Egyptian mythology, doppelgänger in, 4
animals, and the concept of mind, 8
antiquity, the double in, 18–32
   The Epic of Gilgamesh, 27–29
   Euripides, 18–21
   Loki, 30–32
   Plautus, 21–26
anxiety, autoscopy and, 131
Asylum (McGrath), 91
Athens, classical, 18
autoscopic hallucination, 13, 128
   comparison of literary examples with clinical psychopathology, 51
   the concept of, 14
   in Dostoyevsky's *The Double*, 51
   in Dostoyevsky's *The Insulted and The Injured*, 54
   the experience of, 51
   vs. heautoscopy proper, 14
   in Hoffmann's *The Devil's Elixir*, 43
   in Maupassant's 'The Horla', 58
   in Nabokov's *Despair*, 103
   perception of the simulacrum, 38
autoscopy, 11
   and anxiety, 131
   Cartesian duality and, 132
   in clinical psychopathology, 13–15
   concept of, 13
   differentiation from out-of-the-body experience, 145–146, 148
   in Dostoyevsky's *The Double*, 56–57
   in Dostoyevsky's *The Insulted and The Injured*, 54
   in Ellis's *Lunar Park*, 75
   the experience of being confronted with one's doppelgänger in, 66
   likely personal experiences, 67
   McConnell's description, 127
   medical conditions occurring in, 131
   migraine and, 131
   neural mechanisms, 131–132, 144
   phenomenology of in Hogg's *Confessions*, 39–40
   and related phenomena, 127–132
   and the debate about the nature of the mind-body relationship, 151
   and the relationship between subject and duplicate, 65–66
   variants, 13, 128
   visual perception in, 142
Avatar (Cameron), 123, 125
Ayoade, Richard, 117

INDEX

The Bacchae (Euripides), 19
Bachman, Richard, *see also* King, Stephen, 72
Baker, Roy Ward, 97
Bass, Saul, 116
Beauchamp, Christine L., 135
Bergman, Ingrid, 113
Bernhardt, Sarah, 138
bildungsroman, meaning of, 1
Blanke, Olaf, investigations into autoscopy and out-of-the-body experience, 144–151
Blindness (Saramago), 61
body, Sergio Moravia on the relationship between mind and, 7–8
body image
 vs. body schema, 155
 malleability, 155
 and phantom limbs in amputees, 156
 Schilder's work, 155
 social and cultural dimensions, 155
Borges, Jorge Luis
 'Borges and I', 75–76
 'The Other', 76
Bos, E. M., 150
Bradbury, Ray
 Fahrenheit 451, 88
 Martian Chronicles, 88
 'The Martian', 88–91
brain, mapping function, 157–158
Brodie, William (Deacon Brodie), 81–83
 description of, 82
 double life, 81
 hanging, 83
 R. L. Stevenson's interest, 82
The Brothers Karamazov (Dostoyevsky), 48
The Brothers Menaechmus (Plautus), 24–25, 65
Brugger, P., 128

Caird, Mona, 85
Cameron, James, *Avatar*, 123, 125
Capgras, Jean Marie Joseph, 137
Capgras syndrome, 15, 137–138
 Bradbury's 'The Martian' and, 89, 90
 characteristics, 136
 in McGrath's *Spider*, 94, 96
 in Nabokov's *Despair*, 104
 original name, 24
Cartesian dualism, 8, 15, 132, 152, 162
Celtic culture, fetches in, 4
Christodoulou, George, 139
Churchland, P. M., 154

clinical psychology, the double in, 127–141
clinical psychopathology, the double in, 13–17
 autoscopy and its variants, 13–15
 delusional misidentification syndrome, 15–17
cognition, Gibbs on the meaning of, 10
comedy, 21–23, 24–25, 29, 65, 136, 167
Comero, George A., 73
Costandi, Moheb, 160–162
 The New Science of Self-consciousness: Body Am I, 160
Cotten, Joseph, 107
Courbon, P., 138
Crime and Punishment (Dostoyevsky), 48
Cronenberg, David, 91

Damasio, Antonio, 156–160
 Self Comes to Mind, 156
The Dark Half (King), 47, 71–73
 double motif in, 73
 film adaptation, 73, 117
 plot, 72
 publication, 72
 and the concept of a writer's alter ego, 72
Deacon Brodie, or The Double Life (Stevenson), 81
Dead Souls (Gogol), 51
death, relationship between seeing one's doppelgänger and the imminence of, 71
déja vu experiences, 103
delusion of inanimate doubles, 15, 16, 136
delusion of intermetamorphosis, in Bradbury's 'The Martian', 90
delusional misidentification syndrome, 136–137
 in clinical psychopathology, 15–17
 core idea, 137
 in McGrath's *Spider*, 103
 role of the 'double' concept, 136
 in the Wachowskis's *The Matrix*, 122
delusions of subjective doubles, in Endō's *Scandal*, 69
depersonalization, 14–15, 75, 93
 negative heautoscopy and, 130
depression
 autoscopy and, 131
 Dostoyevsky's experience of, 52–53
 inner heautoscopy and, 131
 Poe's battles with, 46
 in Saramago's *The Double*, 62

INDEX

depression (cont.)
William Sharp's experience of, 86
Descartes, René, theory of dualism, *see also* Cartesian dualism, 8, 152
Despair (Nabokov), 97–104
   autoscopic hallucination in, 103
   Capgras syndrome in, 104
   central role of identity in, 101
   comparison with Saramago's *The Double*, 101
   dissociation in, 101–102
   Hermann's preoccupation with mirrors, 103
   manifestation of the double motif, 100, 102
   narrative structure, 99
The Devil's Elixir (Hoffmann), 41, 45
   autoscopic hallucination in, 43
   feeling of presence in, 43
   similarities and connections with Hogg's *Confessions*, 44–45
Diary of a Madman (Gogol), 57
Die Serapionsbrüder (*The Serapion Brethren*) (Hoffmann), 41
The Discovery of the Unconscious (Ellenberger), 133
disembodiment
   defined, 145
   distinguishing from spatial localization and visual spatial perspective, 145
   vestibular dysfunction and, 146
dissociation
   association with traumatic experiences in childhood, 102
   in McGrath's *Spider*, 92–93
   in Nabokov's *Despair*, 101–102
dissociative amnesia, 133
dissociative identity disorder (multiple personality disorder), 17, 132–135
   Christine Beauchamp's case, 135
   Eberhardt Gmelin's case, 134
   historical perspective, 133, 140
   in Hitchcock's *Psycho*, 115–117
   Mary Reynolds case, 133
   R. L. Stevenson's anticipation of the phenomenology, 81
   Stevenson's *Jekyll and Hyde* as literary exemplar of, 101
Don Quixote, relationship between Sancho Panza and, 29
doppelgänger
   birth of a tradition, 3
   the experience of being confronted with one's, 66
   first use of the term, 1
   Meehan's analysis, 3
   related concepts in cultural groups, 4
   translation, 1
Dostoyevsky, Fyodor, 47–57
   The Brothers Karamazov, 48
   Crime and Punishment, 48
   The Double, 49–51
   epilepsy, 48, 52–53, 56
   experience of depression, 52–53
   Hoffmann's influence, 45
   The Idiot, 48, 53–54
   The Insulted and The Injured, 54
   likely personal experience of autoscopy, 67
   most famous works, 48
   Notes from Underground, 48
   The Possessed, 54
the double
   experiences encountered in clinical psychiatry, 7
   in literature, 33, 76–77
   in neuroscience, 142
The Double (Ayoade), 117
The Double (Dostoyevsky), 49–51
   autoscopic hallucination in, 58
   Borges's discussion of, 76
   feeling of presence in, 33, 50–51
   film adaptation, 117
   Hitchcock's familiarity with, 110
   plot, 49
   publication, 49
The Double (Saramago), 61–67, 70
   comparison with Nabokov's *Despair*, 101
   depression in, 62
   feeling of presence in, 62–63
   film adaptation, 117
double motif
   in Bradbury's 'The Martian', 97
   cinematic history, 117, 125–126
   cinematographic resources deployed in depicting, 117
   in Endō's *Scandal*, 68–69
   Hitchcock as best exponent of, 106
   in Hitchcock's *Psycho*, 114, 115
   in Hitchcock's *Shadow of a Doubt*, 108
   in Hitchcock's *Strangers on a Train*, 108, 109
   importance in popular culture, 16, 137, 152

INDEX

in King's *The Dark Half*, 73
in literature vs. in psychopathology, 31
in Nabokov's *Despair*, 100, 102
in Richter's *Siebenkäs*, 1
in sci-fi films, 117
in the Wachowskis's *The Matrix*, 122
Dreyer, Carl, *The Passion of Joan of Arc*, 112
dualism, Descartes's theory, *see also* Cartesian dualism, 8
duality
   Karl Miller on the function of, 38
   the notion of in fiction, 78
   role of in fiction, 78–87
   of the human body, 4
duplication, preoccupation with the notion of, 4

egocentric mental transformations, vs. allocentric, 149
Electra (Euripides), 19
Ellenberger, H. F., 133
   The Discovery of the Unconscious, 133
   on Eberhardt Gmelin's case, 134
Ellis, Bret Easton
   American Psycho, 74, 75
   Less Than Zero, 74
   Lunar Park, 47, 71, 74–75
embodiment, 10–11, 33, 150, 154, 158–159
Embodiment and Cognitive Science (Gibbs Jr), 10–11, 158
empirical literature, importance of, 11–13
Endō, Shūsaku, 47
   Scandal, 67–71
   Shame, 140
   Silence, 67
   themes of works, 67–68
Enemy (Villeneuve), 117
The Epic of Gilgamesh (circa 1700 BC), 27–29
   as depiction of 'the opposing self', 29
   likely origins, 27
   story of Enkidu, 28–29
   story of Gilgamesh, 27–28
   and the resolution of conflict, 29
epilepsy
   autoscopy and, 131
   Dostoyevsky's experience of, 48, 52–53
   Dostoyevsky's portrayal of, 56
   role in out-of-the-body or autoscopic experience, 14, 146
Espenschied, Lloyd, 111
Euripides
   Alcestis, 19

The Bacchae, 19
   the double in, 18–21
Electra, 19
Helen, 19–21
Hippolytus, 19
Medea, 19
   plays of, 18–19
The Women of Troy, 19
experiential double, distinction between ideational double and, 32
extra-personal space, 146–147

facial recognition, fragility of identity by way of, 16, 137
Fahrenheit 451 (Bradbury), 88
Fail, G., 138
Falconetti, Renee, 112
The Fall of the House of Usher (Poe), 45
feeling of presence, 13, 128
   in Dostoyevsky's *The Double*, 33, 50, 51
   in Dostoyevsky's *The Possessed*, 54
   in Ellis's *Lunar Park*, 75
   the experience of, 129
   in Hoffmann's *The Devil's Elixir*, 43
   Lukianowicz's description, 129
   in Maupassant's 'The Horla', 58
   in Saramago's *The Double*, 62–63
fetches
   in Celtic culture, 4
   in Icelandic sagas, 4
   in Norse sagas, 71
Fishburne, Laurence, 121
Flegeljahre (Richter), 1
Fleming, Victor, 97
Fonda, Henry, 110
Frégoli, Leopoldo, 30, 31, 139
Frégoli syndrome, 30, 89, 139
   comparison with syndrome of intermetamorphosis, 136
Freud, Sigmund, 133
fylgja (fetch in Icelandic sagas), 4

Gaeta, John, 122
The Ghost of One's Self (Meehan), 3
Gibbs, Raymond, *Embodiment and Cognitive Science*, 10–11, 158
Gmelin, Eberhardt, 134
Gogol, Nikolai
   Dead Souls, 51
   Diary of a Madman, 57
Gorenshtein, Fridrikh, 120
Groat, William B., 111

INDEX

guilt
    in Hitchcock's *Psycho*, 115
    in Hitchcock's *Strangers on a Train*, 109

Head, Henry, 155
head injury
    and negative heautoscopy, 130, 131
    and out-of-the-body experience, 129–130
heautoscopy proper, 14, 128
    vs. autoscopic hallucination, 14
    comparison of literary examples with clinical psychopathology, 51
    the concept of, 14
    in Dostoyevsky's *The Double*, 51
    the experience of, 51, 128–129
    Lhermitte's description, 128
    visual perception in, 142
Hedren, Tippi, 113
Helen (Euripides), 19–21
    the encounter of Helen and Menelaus, 21
    function of the double in, 20
    Helen as mirror image, 21
    ideational double in, 19
Highsmith, Patricia, 110
Hippolytus (Euripides), 19
His Dark Materials (Pullman), 4
Hitchcock, Alfred, 106–117
    The 39 Steps, 106
    as best exponent of the double motif, 106
    comparison between women and suspense, 114
    early films, 106
    The Lodger, 106
    Notorious, 106
    obsession with the dress and demeanour of his leading ladies, 113
    Psycho, 106, 114–117
    Shadow of a Doubt, 106, 107–108
    Strangers on a Train, 106, 108–110
    Vertigo, 106, 112–114
    The Wrong Man, 106, 110–112
Hitchcock, Patricia, 110, 115
Hoffmann, E. T. A., 1, 71
    The Devil's Elixir, 41–45
    influence on Hogg's *Confessions*, 41
    influence on other writers, 45
    works of, 41
Hogg, James, 71
    comparison of approach with Dostoyevsky and Maupassant, 36, 39
    Hoffmann's influence, 41
    Karl Miller's description, 41
    likely personal experience of autoscopy, 67
    most famous poems, 34
    The Private Memoirs and Confessions of a Justified Sinner, 34–41
human language, embodiment and, 10
Hume, David, *A Treatise of Human Nature*, 9–10
Hutton, Timothy, 73

Icelandic sagas, fetches in, 4
ideational double, 13
    distinction between experiential double and, 32
identical doubles, literary function, 29
identical twins
    in Plautus's *The Brothers Menaechmus*, 24–25
    Romulus and Remus, 26
    Stephen King on, 73
    and the physical uniqueness of persons, 16–17, 66
    unsettling nature of encounters with, 25
identity
    central role in the Nabokov's *Despair*, 101
    exploration of in the Wachowskis's *The Matrix*, 122
    fragility by way of facial recognition, 16, 137
Identity, Consciousness and Value (Unger), 12–13
identity theories, 153
    varieties of, 153
The Idiot (Dostoyevsky), 48, 53–54
Illusion de Sosie, 24
The Image and Appearance of the Human Body (Schilder), 154–156
implicit notion, 88
inanimate doubles, delusion of, 15, 16, 136
inner autoscopy, 14, 128
inner heautoscopy
    the concept of, 15
    and depression, 131
    the experience of, 131
    Rao's description, 131
inner life of the writer
    in Ellis's *Lunar Park*, 74–75
    in Endō's *Scandal*, 68
    in Hitchcock's *Vertigo*, 113–114
    in King's *The Dark Half*, 72–73
The Insulted and The Injured (Dostoyevsky), 54

INDEX

intermetamorphosis, syndrome of, 15–16, 136
It (King), 72

Jamais vu experiences, 103
Janet, Pierre, 102, 133
Jung, Carl Gustav, 133

Kafka, Franz, Hoffmann's influence, 45
Kelly, Grace, 113
Kidnapped (Stevenson), 79
Kim's, Jaegwon, 153
King, Stephen, 47, 71
   The Dark Half, 47, 71, 72–73
   on identical twins, 73
   It, 72
   Misery, 72
   most famous and influential works, 72
   Pet Sematary, 72
   pseudonym, 72
   The Shining, 72
   The Stand, 72

The Lady Vanishes (Hitchcock), 106
Lang, Fritz, 117
   Metropolis, 117
Lang, Stephen, 124
latent double, distinction between manifest double and, 31
Leigh, Janet, 115
Lem, Stanislaw, *Solaris*, 118–120
Less Than Zero (Ellis), 74
The Lodger (Hitchcock), 106
Lolita (Nabokov), 98
Lopez, C., 150
Lukianowicz, N., 129
Lunar Park (Ellis), 47, 71, 74–75
   autobiographical elements, 74
   blurring of boundaries between fiction and reality, 74
   feeling of presence in, 75
   plot, 74
   publication, 74
Lunn, V., 129

Macleod, Fiona
   works, 84
   see also Sharp, William.
Mamoulian, Rouben, 97
The Man Who Was Jekyll and Hyde (Wilson), 82
manifest double
   distinction between latent double and, 31

in Hogg's *Confessions*, 35–36, 40
Martian Chronicles (Bradbury), 88
matricide, in McGrath's *Spider*, 96
The Matrix (Wachowskis), 120–123
   cinema technology employed in, 122
   delusional misidentification syndrome in, 122
   double motifs, 122
   exploration of identity in, 122
   impact on popular culture, 122
   Paul Meehan on, 123
   sequels, 122
The Matrix Reloaded (Wachowskis), 123
Maupassant, Guy de, 57–61, 106
   likely personal experience of autoscopy, 67
   'The Horla', 58–61
McConnell, W. B., 127
McGinn, C., 153
McGrath, Patrick
   Asylum, 91
   Spider, 91–97
McLeod, Fiona, William Sharp and, *see also* Sharp, William, 83–86
Meehan, Paul, 3
   on Cameron's *Avatar*, 125
   The Ghost of One's Self, 3
   on Tarkovsky's *Solaris*, 120
   on the Wachowskis's *Matrix* films, 123
meeting of doubles
   in Dostoyevsky's *The Double*, 50
   in Endō's *Scandal*, 70
   in Hitchcock's *Strangers on a Train*, 109
   in Hitchcock's *The Wrong Man*, 111
   in Richter's *Siebenkäs*, 2–3
Melzack, R., 143
Merleau-Ponty, Maurice, *Phenomenology of Perception*, 160
Metropolis (Lang), 117
migraine, autoscopy and, 131
Miles, Vera, 110, 113
Miller, Karl, 38
   on Hoffmann's influence on other writers, 45
   on James Hogg, 41
   on R. L. Stevenson, 81
mind
   the concept of self and, 7–10
   Gilbert Ryle's thesis, 8
   philosophical theories' reliance on imaginary cases, 12

INDEX

mind–body relationship, Sergio Moravia on, 7–8
mirror image, Euripides's Helen as, 21
mirrors
   Hermann's preoccupation with in Nabokov's *Despair*, 103
   symbolism of in Hitchcock's *Psycho*, 115
Misery (King), 72
mistaken identity
   in Hitchcock's *The Wrong Man*, 110, 111
   in Plautus's *Amphitryron*, 24–25, 136
Mitchill, S. L., 133
Molière, Plautus's influence on, 23
Moravia, Sergio, on the relationship between mind and body, 7–8
Moss, Carrie-Anne, 121
Mountain Lovers (Macleod), 84

Nabokov, Vladimir
   Despair, 97–104
   early life, 97
   Lolita, 98
Nakul, E., 150
Narcissus, Robert Rogers on the myth of, 21
negative autoscopy, 14
   in Maupassant's 'The Horla', 58, 60
negative heautoscopy
   the concept of, 15
   the experience of, 130
   head injury and, 130–131
   Lunn's description, 130–131
   in Maupassant's 'The Horla', 130
neural mechanisms
   of autoscopy, 131–132, 144
   of out-of-the-body experience, 144–145
neuromatrix, Melzack's notion, 143
neuronal networks, as a kind of neural double of the body, 156
neuroscience
   aim of the project, 154
   the double in, 142
The New Science of Self-consciousness: Body Am I (Costandi), 160
non-identical double, literary function, 29
Norse mythology
   fetches in, 4, 71
   Loki, 30–31
   vardogers, 4
Notes from Underground (Dostoyevsky), 48
Notorious (Hitchcock), 106
Novak, Kim, 112–113

O'Connor, Frank, 111
'The Opposing Self', Robert Rogers's notion, 29
Ormonde, Czenzi, 110
'The Other' (Borges), 76
other, the double as, 33, 76–77
otolith dysfunction, role in out-of-the-body experience, 146
out-of-the-body experience, 14, 64, 128
   components, 145
   the concept of, 14
   differentiation from autoscopy, 145–146, 148
   the experience of, 129
   head injury and, 129–130
   Lunn's description, 129–130
   neural mechanisms, 144–145
   role of otolith dysfunction, 146
   visual perception in, 142
Oyebode, F., 132

pain, subjective experience of, 152
parasomatic body, 146
Parkinson's disease, 12
The Passion of Joan of Arc (Dreyer), 112
Peloponnesian War, 18
'perdurable empathy', and the resolution of conflict, 29
personal identity
   exploring the nature of with imaginary examples, 12–13
   Kathleen Wilkes on, 13
personal space, 146–147
Pet Sematary (King), 72
phantom limbs
   amputees, 156
   children with congenitally absent limbs, 143
   role of neuronal networks, 157
Pharais (Macleod), 84
Phenomenology of Perception (Merleau-Ponty), 160
phocomelia, 143
Plautus, Titus Maccius, 21–26, 142
   Amphitryon, 23–24, 136
   The Brothers Menaechmus, 24–25, 65
   influence on European literature, 23
Poe, Edgar Allan
   battles with depression, 46
   The Fall of the House of Usher, 45
   most famous works, 45
   'William Wilson', 45–47, 110

INDEX

writing style, 45
The Possessed (Dostoyevsky), 54
possession, dissociative personality and, 133
posture, body image and, 155, 156
Prince, Morton, on Christine Beauchamp's case, 135
The Private Memoirs and Confessions of a Justified Sinner (Hogg), 34–41
  manifest double in, 35–36, 40
  phenomenology of autoscopy in, 39–40
  similarities and connections with Hoffmann's *Devil's Elixir*, 44–45
proprioception, 11, 143, 159, 162
Prose Edda (Sturluson), 31
Proteus
  Hogg's comparison of the double concept with, 37–38
  variant of in Bradbury's 'The Martian', 89
Psycho (Hitchcock), 106, 114–117
  dissociative identity disorder in, 115–117
  double motif in, 114, 115
  as filmic update of R. L. Stevenson's *Jekyll and Hyde*, 117
  guilt in, 115
  symbolism of mirrors, 115
  title designs, 116
Pullman, Philip, *His Dark Materials*, 4

The Raven (Poe), 45
Rayment, Neil & Adrian, 123
Real People (Wilkes), 13
Reboul-Lachaux, Jean, 137
reduplicative paramnesia, 15–16, 75, 122, 136
Reeves, Keanu, 121
reputational damage, association of the name Helen with, 20
Reynolds, Mary, 133
Ribisi, Giovanni, 124
Richter, Jean Paul
  self-consciousness, 2
  Siebenkäs, 1–3
Rinder, Edith Wingate, 84–85
Robertson, John S., 97
Robine, Gabrielle, 138
Rogers, Robert, 21
  preoccupation with psychoanalytic investigation of the double in literature, 31
  on the distinction between manifest and latent doubles, 31
  on the relationship between Don Quixote and Sancho Panza, 29
Romero, George, 117
Romulus and Remus, 26
Ryle, Gilbert, on the concept of mind, 8

Saldaña, Zoë, 124
Saramago, José, 47
  Blindness, 61
  The Double, 61–67, 70
Scandal (Endō), 67, 71
  delusions of subjective doubles in, 69
  double motif, 68–69
  materialization and agency of the doppelgänger, 69–70
  meeting of doubles in, 70
  plot and setting, 68
  and the writer's inner life, 68
Schilder, Paul
  The Image and Appearance of the Human Body, 154–156
  on phantom limbs in amputees, 156
schizophrenia, autoscopy and, 131
Scott, Gordon, 112
self
  as composite of different perceptual modalities, 162
  the concept of mind and, 7–10
  link to tactile-kinaesthetic activity, 11
  and loss of material from the brain, 12–13
  relationship to the body, 161–162
  role of embodiment in creating a sense of, 11
  singular nature of, 5–6
Self Comes to Mind (Damasio), 156
self-consciousness, Richter on, 2
self-deception, exploration of in Nabokov's *Despair*, 101
self-location, role of the temporo-parietal junction, 145, 148
sense of self
  creation of, 153
  creation role of embodiment, 11
  dissociative identity disorder and, 135
  pillars, 5
  Schilder's examination of, 154
Shadow of a Doubt (Hitchcock), 106, 107–108
Shakespeare, William, Plautus's influence on, 23
Shame (Endō), 140
shape-shifting, 30–31
Sharp, Elizabeth, 85

INDEX

Sharp, Mary, 85
Sharp, William
  experience of depression, 86
  and Fiona McLeod, 83–86
The Shining (King), 72
Siebenkäs (Richter), 1–3
  double motif, 1
  meeting of doubles in, 2–3
  plot, 1
Silence (Endō), 67
Solaris (Lem), 118–120
  comparison with Tarkovsky's film adaptation, 119–120
  story and themes, 118–119
Solaris (Tarkovsky), 119–120
  Paul Meehan on, 120
somnambulistic possession, 133
Sophocles, 18
Spider (McGrath)
  Capgras syndrome in, 94, 96
  delusional misidentification syndrome in, 103
  dissociation in, 92–93
  expression of the double motif, 97
  implicit notion of the double, 100
  matricide in, 96
  unreliable narrators in, 91–92
Spoto, Donald
  on Hitchcock's ability to respond to women, 114
  on Hitchcock's familiarity with the double motif in literature, 110
  on Hitchcock's *Shadow of a Doubt*, 108
  on Hitchcock's *Strangers on a Train*, 110
  on symbolism in Hitchcock's *Psycho*, 116
  on the relationship between Hitchcock and Vera Miles, 112
  on the relevance of Hitchcock's biography for *Vertigo*, 113
The Stand (King), 72
Stevenson, Robert Louis, 127
  anticipation of dissociative identity disorder, 81
  Deacon Brodie, or The Double Life, 81
  interest in William Brodie, 82
  Karl Miller on, 81
  notable works, 79
  The Strange Case of Dr Jekyll and Mr Hyde, 33, 78–83
Stewart, James, 112–113
The Strange Case of Dr Jekyll and Mr Hyde (Stevenson), 33, 78–83
  comparison with McGrath's *Spider*, 100
  comparison with Nabokov's *Despair*, 100, 102
  on film, 97
  Hitchcock's *Psycho* as filmic update of, 117
  as literary exemplar of dissociative identity disorder, 101
Strangers on a Train (Hitchcock), 106, 108–110
  double motif in, 108, 109
  guilt in, 109
  meeting of doubles in, 109
  source of adaptation, 110
Strawson, Galen, 9
The Student of Prague (Wegener), 117
Sturluson, Snorri, 31
subjective doubles, syndrome of, 15–16, 136, 139–140
superior colliculus, mapping function, 158
syndrome of intermetamorphosis, 15–16, 136
syndrome of subjective doubles, 15–16, 139–140
  characteristics, 136

tactile-kinaesthetic activity, 11, 159
Tarkovsky, Andrei, *Solaris*, 118–120
Taylor, Ronald, introduction to his translation of Hoffmann's *The Devil's Elixir*, 44
The Tell-Tale Heart (Poe), 45
temporo-parietal junction
  association with out-of-the-body experiences and autoscopy, 145–146, 150
  role of in self-location, 145, 148
  role of in spatial perception and body representation, 131
'The Horla' (Maupassant), 58–61
  autoscopic hallucination in, 51, 56–57
  negative autoscopy in, 58, 60
  negative heautoscopy in, 130
'The Martian' (Bradbury), 88–91
  Capgras syndrome in, 89, 90
  delusion of intermetamorphosis in, 90
  expression of the double motif, 97
thought experiments, 12, 13
Titan (Richter), 1
token identity theory, 153
traumatic brain injury, autoscopy and, 131

Travels with a Donkey in the Cevennes and In the South Seas (Stevenson), 79
Treasure Island (Stevenson), 79, 81
A Treatise of Human Nature (Hume & Selby-Bigge), 9–10
type identity theory, 153

Unger, Peter, *Identity, Consciousness and Value*, 12–13
unique self, subjective experience, 5–6
unreliable narrators
  in McGrath's *Spider*, 91–92
  in Nabokov's *Despair*, 98, 99, 100, 104
  in Nabokov's *Lolita*, 98
unsettling feelings, encounters with doubles and, 25

Vertigo (Hitchcock), 106, 112–114
  Donald Spoto on the relevance of Hitchcock's biography, 113
  personal drama behind the scenes, 112
  plot, 112
  themes explored in, 113
vestibular processing, contribution to disintegration of bodily information, 150

Villeneuve, Denis, 117
virtual self, creation of, 160
vision, the function of, 160
visual hallucinations, in Dostoyevsky's *The Possessed*, 54
visual perception, in autoscopy, 142

Wachowskis, *The Matrix*, 120–123
The Washer of the Ford (Macleod), 84
Weaver, Sigourney, 124
Whitman, Walt, 18
Wilkes, Kathleen, *Real People*, 13
'William Wilson' (Poe), 45–47, 110
Wilson, Rick, *The Man Who Was Jekyll and Hyde*, 82
The Women of Troy (Euripides), 19
Worthington, Sam, 124
Wright, Teresa, 107
The Wrong Man (Hitchcock), 106, 111–112
  factual basis, 110–111
  meeting of doubles in, 111
  personal drama behind the scenes, 112
  plot, 111

Yoruba, 4
Yusov, Vadim, 120

For EU product safety concerns, contact us at Calle de José Abascal, 56–1°,
28003 Madrid, Spain or eugpsr@cambridge.org.

www.ingramcontent.com/pod-product-compliance
Lightning Source LLC
LaVergne TN
LVHW021715060526
838200LV00050B/2684